Life is Terminal:
A Doctor's Common Sense
Guide for Making it to

The End

Arthur H. Parsons M.D.

MOONLIGHT PRESS | TORONTO

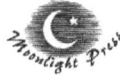

MOONLIGHT PRESS
Toronto, CANADA
www.moonlightpresstoronto.com

DISCLAIMER:
None of the material in this book is intended to provide specific medical or healthcare
advice. This book is not intended as a substitute for the medical advice of physicians or other
healthcare providers. The reader should regularly consult a physician in matters relating to
his/her health and particularly with respect to any symptoms that may require diagnosis or
medical attention. Neither the author nor the publisher, or other representatives will be
liable for damages arising out of or in connection with the use of this book.

For information

moonlightpressinfo@gmail.com

ISBN 978-0-9958882-0-3

OTHER BOOKS BY ARTHUR PARSONS

Patient Power! The Smart Patient's Guide to Health Care
University of Toronto Press (with Patricia Parsons)

*When Older is Wiser: A Guide to Healthcare Decisions for Older
Adults and their Families*
Doubleday Canada (with Patricia Parsons)

Health Care Ethics. Wall and Emerson, Inc. (with Patricia Parsons)

Hippocrates Now! Is Your Doctor Ethical?
University of Toronto Press (with Patricia Parsons)

CONTENTS

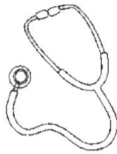

Life should be perceived as positive until it isn't,
rather than potentially negative until it is.

~ A.H. Parsons M.D.

IN THE BEGINNING

PETE KOWALSKI HESITATED BRIEFLY as he placed his hand on the smooth glass door. He looked at the sign and took a deep breath. Just below the names "Dr. Anthony Kramer" and "Dr. Sherrilynne Fontaine" and just above "Family Medicine & Obstetrics," was "Dr. Peter Kowalski."

"This is it," he thought. "Real people think I'm a real doctor." He shifted the large box containing his framed medical degree and a few other personal items to decorate his office so he could free up a hand to open the door.

He wondered if, thirty-five years from now, he'd still remember this moment – the moment just before he stepped into his own office for his very first day as a family physician. He just hoped that the past years of hard work had been enough – enough for him to know what to do, and perhaps equally important, what to say.

He stepped into the main reception area where the clock on the wall told him it was five minutes before eight. The patient waiting area was empty as was the reception desk. But he could hear voices down one of the halls.

"Good morning, Dr. Kowalski," came a bright voice, startling him out of his reverie.

He turned quickly.

"Welcome to your new office."

A happy-looking fortysomething woman, Tara Kasapolous had worked for Dr. Kramer for more than fifteen years. Pete had met her when he spent some time

1

here in the office during a rotation when he was a medical student. It was that experience that had convinced him his calling was to be a family physician. He had wanted nothing more than to join Dr. Kramer and Dr. Fontaine in their practice. Pete followed her into the staff lunch room.

"I suppose you'll be wanting to see your new digs," she said, pouring two cups of coffee.

"Sure," Pete said, feeling a bit out of place as the new kid on the block. Dr. Kramer had renovated the office to accommodate Pete who had yet to see the finished product.

"Is Dr. Kramer here yet?" he asked sipping from the cup of coffee in his free hand.

"Dr. K.? Of course. He starts seeing patients at 7:15 right after rounds at the hospital to see his new mothers and babies. He's already seen three patients this morning."

Pete was feeling tired already. *I'll have to start going to bed earlier*, he was thinking. Tara was beaming at him. She clearly loved her work and seemed to enjoy letting Pete know about Dr. Kramer's schedule even after over twenty years of practice.

"This way," she said, gesturing down the hall past Dr. Kramer's waiting room. "Dr. Fontaine doesn't come in until after noon on Mondays. She works all night in the emergency room."

Pete followed her into his bright, new office space. It wasn't large, but he would make it his own before too long.

"You make yourself comfortable. Your first patient is at 8:45. I'll get you her chart." She left him sitting at his desk with his coffee, contemplating his day ahead.

Pete settled into the chair with his coffee pondering what was ahead. What kinds of patients awaited him? What kinds of problems would they have? Would he really be able to help them? And all of this on his first day on the job. He wouldn't be left alone for long to ponder.

~

Elizabeth Michaud hadn't been sleeping well for the past few weeks. As she pulled her little car into a parking space outside Dr. Kramer's office building, she caught sight of her reflection in the rear-view mirror.

"I look like hell," she said out loud to the empty car.

At only 47, she ought to look better, she was thinking. At least that's what her husband had told her this very morning at breakfast. She knew it, too. She hadn't felt the same since that car accident a year ago when she hurt her back. And now she was a mess. What was worse, when she had called Dr. Kramer's office yesterday to make an appointment, Tara had told her she'd have to wait a week and a half for an appointment with Dr. Kramer or see someone called Dr. Kowalski, the new guy. Elizabeth had settled for seeing Dr. Kowalski, but now she was having second thoughts. How could some new hot shot doctor know anything at all about being a middle-aged mother of three whose life was falling apart?

She heaved herself out of the car thinking, I suppose I should lose a bit of weight, but what for? She sighed and went into the office building. She took the elevator to the third floor and announced herself at the desk. She settled heavily into the nearest seat absently picking up a fitness magazine on the table beside her.

When Sylvia, the new nurse that Dr. Kramer had hired to assist Pete, ushered Elizabeth into his private office fifteen minutes later, Pete had already begun to make the office his own. Elizabeth noticed that there was a brass bell on the desk and wondered if it was there for patients to ring if he took too long getting to them. Behind his head hung his medical degree, or at least she suspected that it was. Since it was written in Latin, she couldn't really be sure, but it looked official. Beside the diploma was a small piece of paper framed in brass. She peered at it closely, delaying the moment when she would be compelled to take stock of this young man before her and divulge her most intimate secrets.

The frame contained a tiny quote. It read: "There is only one good, knowledge, and one evil, ignorance. Socrates."

God, she thought. Save me from philosophical doctors.

"Mrs. Michaud?" Pete said as he extended his hand to her.

Elizabeth shook his hand weakly.

"I'm Dr. Kowalski," he said brightly, "but feel free to call me Pete if it makes you more comfortable."

"Dr. Kowalski will be fine," she said, clasping her hands tightly in her lap as she sat there looking across the desk at him. He was awfully nice looking – disconcertingly so, she thought. There was a time when she would have enjoyed a conversation with a handsome doctor, but now the prospect made her uncomfortable.

"I understand you've been seeing Dr. Kramer for some years now." He looked at the computer screen on his desk. "What brings you to the office today?"

"I need you to do something to make me sleep better."

"Uh-huh," Pete murmured as he glanced quickly down the list he had written out from his brief perusal of her chart. Forty-seven-year old married mother, slightly obese. Dr. Kramer had delivered her three children who were all normal at birth, the youngest now ten years old. Over the past decade she had been arriving in the office increasingly frequently with a series of non-specific complaints. Last year she had been rear-ended while her car was stopped at a stop sign, and her lawyer had been pursuing insurance money from the people who hit her ever since. Dr. Kramer had tried to help her with her back pain, but her lawyer had kept encouraging her to document every twinge. (*It must be difficult to try to recover when you're being told to focus on your pain*, Peter was thinking.) Her weight had started to climb, and her oldest daughter, now fifteen, had had a difficult year at school dealing with what she perceived as her own weight problem for which she evidently blamed her mother. All of this history was documented in Dr. Kramer's charted notes.

The woman sitting before him looked drawn and pale.

"Oh, yes," she added, "and I need you to do something about my headaches."

Mrs. Michaud was Pete's third patient this morning and each one of them, in their own way, had said the same thing. "I need *you* to do something." *Each of them wanted Pete to fix them.*

~

Dr. Kowalski had seemed nice enough, Elizabeth thought as she took the elevator down to the ground floor on her way to the pharmacy to have her prescription filled. She wasn't at all sure, however, about his plan to have her return to see him in a week. Surely, she could decide if she needed to see a doctor. But he hadn't given her as large a prescription for sleeping pills as she had wanted. In fact, he hadn't wanted to give her the prescription at all, only doing so after she promised to come back in a week. Now she didn't have a choice.

As she stood in line at the pharmacy counter waiting for her little bottle of pills, the older woman in front of her turned to speak.

"It's a lovely day, isn't it?"

The woman smiled at Elizabeth who realized that she hadn't noticed the weather at all. In fact, she hadn't noticed anything at all today except herself it seemed.

"Yes," she said anyway, "I suppose it is."

Elizabeth was feeling distracted. She wasn't at all sure she wanted to launch into a conversation with a complete stranger.

"It's peculiar, isn't it," the woman continued, "Everyone stands here clutching their little pieces of paper waiting for their magic pills and potions. When all we really need is to have more pleasure in our lives."

Elizabeth didn't say a word. She was looking at the twinkle in the woman's eyes. They were old eyes to be sure, with lines radiating out from the creases, yet something about them seemed young. They seemed to have a depth of experience, but there was also a clarity suggesting an ability to see things anew. *Lucky her,* Elizabeth thought. *Retired, happy, well-heeled, healthy. Lucky her.*

The woman was wearing a jaunty red beret perched rakishly on the silver curls that curved out around the rim. She had flung the matching scarf haphazardly around her neck making one think that she must have thrown it there with a smile and a wink.

"Your scarf is nice," Elizabeth said to her.

"Thank-you, dear," she said, winking. "A red scarf would look devastating on you, you know."

Devastating? thought Elizabeth. *When have I ever been devastating in my entire life?*

The woman reached the pharmacy counter. She didn't seem to be having a prescription filled at all. The young man behind the counter leaned across and she kissed him on the cheek. Then turning to wave at Elizabeth, she was gone.

"You're a friendly pharmacist," Elizabeth said to the young man who began to redden.

"Oh," he said. "She's kind of adopted me as the grandson she never had. A few times a week she comes in, stands in line and tells me she's having a great day. I always feel better for the rest of the day after she's been here." He looked after the departing red scarf and smiled. "She's dying of cancer, you know." Then he turned back to Elizabeth. "How can I help you today, Ma'am?"

Elizabeth was startled. "Cancer?" she said quietly. "She looks so healthy."

"She's a remarkable woman," the pharmacist said. "Now, how can I help you?"

"How about sharing some of that good feeling," she said almost to herself.

"Excuse me?" he said.

"Oh, I have a prescription here," she said absently.

"Have a seat," said the young man. "It'll only be about ten minutes."

Elizabeth sat down to wait again, thinking about her life and her sore back. I guess I should write it down for my lawyer, she was thinking. It'll never get better at this rate.

CHAPTER ONE

THE "COMMON SENSE APPROACH"

*"Nothing is more fairly distributed than common sense –
no one needs more of it than one already has."*
~ Renee Descartes

ASK ANY TEACHER – COMMON SENSE doesn't seem to be all that common these days. In fact, we seem to be suffering from a distinct dearth of anything resembling common sense – or at least knowledge about how and when to apply it.

All you need to do is watch the news each evening or read your favourite online news source. The stories are full of situations that make you want to scratch your head and ask: Where was their common sense?

Consider the following news story. The residents of a small community have just been told that they must boil their drinking water as a result of finding particularly unpleasant bacteria in the local wells. This is the story lead, but as you read further, it becomes clear that the residents have known about the contamination for several years. Several residents have told the newspaper reporter about skin and stomach problems that they have long attributed to drinking the water, but nowhere in the story does it ever become apparent that the residents thought to stop drinking the water. Instead, they complained to the local municipality, but didn't stop using their water until somebody else told them they had to boil it first. This was a classic case of individuals failing to use their common sense which would have allowed them to take responsibility for their own health. Instead, they chose to make it someone else's problem. Consequently, they put up with ill health for much longer than seemed to have been necessary. And, after practicing family medicine for some 45 years, I can attest to the fact that these kinds of problems appeared in my office every day.

But before we can jump right into the heart of using your common sense to assist you in making good decisions about your health (and your life), we need to take a giant step back to make sure we're all talking about the same thing.

So, what *is* health, anyway?

Everybody thinks they know what health is. You probably do too. You probably refer to your health. People ask you how your health is. You remark on other people's health. But have you ever stopped to consider what it is you really mean? When you talk to your doctor, your family or your friends about your health, to what are you referring?

Consider this: A fortyish woman with three children, unfulfilled dreams, a cranky husband, isn't sleeping well and has no apparent illness. She is hardly able to get through her day; she's so fatigued and unhappy. On the other hand, a seventyish woman with terminal cancer, who has decided to live her life to the fullest to the end is enjoying every moment of her remaining months. She occasionally feels what others might term "unwell." She has pain which she treats with the medication she has been given, but she decides to sow happiness wherever she goes and to do some things she never got around to. Which of these women is healthier? And which of them would you prefer to be?

If we define health as the opposite of disease – i.e. the absence of disease -- then clearly, by definition, our younger woman is healthy and our older woman is not. But that hardly tells the whole story.

In fact, most people immediately think about disease whenever they think they are thinking about health. Indeed, our healthcare system is really a disease-care system, isn't it? When was the last time you consulted a *healthcare* provider (doctor, nurse, physiotherapist etc.) because you felt in good health and wanted to learn to stay that way? If you have, good for you, but I know that you are in a tiny minority, and these days with healthcare resources often in limited supply, it can feel immoral to do so. There seem to be so many sick people who need care. So, determining what health means to you is the first step toward defining how you might get to that state and stay there. After all, if you don't know where you're going, how will you ever know when you get there? And if you don't know where you're going, you will probably end up somewhere else – some place that you hadn't intended on ending up. You might achieve good health and never even realize it!

In fact, health is really on an individualized continuum.

```
    A                              C
>═══○══════════○══════════○════════>
          B
```

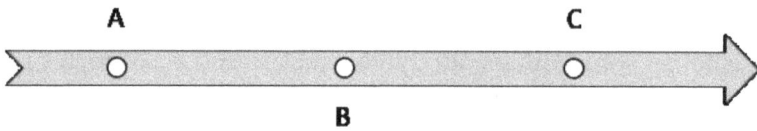

Point A represents *perfect health* (whatever that is – we'll come back to this). Point C represents *complete physical, mental and emotional incapacity*. The important point from a healthcare perspective, however, is point B which is the point at which discernible symptoms arise. The healthcare system's role as we recognize it today generally begins at point B. This means that, theoretically, anywhere on the continuum between point A and point B constitutes an individual's state of health. It's individual because health is something different for everyone (in spite of what the magazines might tell you).

Another less well-known approach to defining health is to define it as a state of "flourishing." The psychology literature has broached this as a way to determine health, but more specifically what they describe as "well-being." Author Tyler VanderWeele (and colleagues) from the Harvard School of Public Health in the US suggest that flourishing concerns "...the full context of what matters in a person's life ... "including,"... more broadly ... relationships, meaning and purpose." This might be worth considering on a personal level.

If we consider the concept of perfect health, and try to understand what that might mean, it soon becomes clear that there really is no such thing. Some artificial, external standard of what it means to be in perfect health is a misguided approach.

There is really no one who is in "perfect health." The fact is that
every human being is going to die someday. It's a bit like the
inscription on a new age tombstone: "Did yoga, ate tofu, died
anyway." And remember, no one has ever been observed to say,
"I wish I had eaten more tofu," as they lay dying.

The most important concept in trying to define what health is
for you is to consider the idea of incapacity. Notice that I indicated
that point C represents *complete physical, mental and emotional
incapacity* – not death. This means that on the continuum between
point B and point C there are degrees of inability to fulfil your
own expectations of what and how your body, mind and spirit
should be. It also means that in some sense you can be healthy
right up until the point of your death.

Consider a 53-year-old man who is unable to accept that his
body is aging. He trains for marathons, water skis with the 20-
year-olds, works out every day, placing his self-imposed physical
challenges before his family responsibilities. Since he is unable to
accept certain inevitabilities of physical change with age, he will
meet his personally-defined level of incapacity much sooner than
other men his age who recognize that aging is a natural process
and choose a balanced life. Think about that. He will meet his
"personally-defined level of incapacity much sooner than other
men his age," when he is seeking precisely the opposite. In other
words, incapacity – or more precisely, when you reach it –
depends on your own expectations about what your health
should be like. People with physical handicaps can be in a state
approaching perfect health if they have realistically set their
expectations and *adapted* their lives to include consideration of
their handicaps.

Thus, your own definition of health may be either a hindrance
to you or a help. Our fifty-something man who refuses to accept
his aging body has set himself up for problems. His definition of
health can do nothing else but get in the way of real, balanced
health.

COMMON SENSE? NOT TOO COMMON, IT SEEMS

- No one lives forever.
- Everyone ages.
- Accidents happen.
- Illness is a fact of the human condition.

You know all these things, and so do most other people who are interested in health. At least you know them intellectually, even though you may not really have accepted them on deeper levels. But the truth is that an important aspect of common sense really means nothing more or less than accepting certain irrefutable truths, and being willing to act on them. Part of common sense is accepting that you won't live forever. The other part is that your life is unlikely as miserable as you may think it is.

American psychologist Nathanial Branden once said, "The first step toward change is awareness; the second step is acceptance." It is this ability to learn to accept sometimes uncomfortable truths – even common sense truths – that is the key to moving forward toward a healthier approach to life's journey.For years it was a common scenario in my office. A patient arrives complaining about the general state of his or her health. Upon further discussion, it emerges that this otherwise sensible person's lifestyle isn't really what we would today consider to be a healthy one. So, I ask the patient this: If I were to provide you with one car that you had to keep for the rest of your life, what kind would it be?

After the patient has fantasized for a moment and come up with a dream choice, I ask this: *Since it is the only car you will ever have, what will you do to ensure that you will still be able to drive this car for many years to come?*

And the litany begins: provide it with the proper fuel and oil, have the oil changed regularly, check the tires, regular servicing, try to avoid driving it in the winter etc. So, then I ask what about this body of yours body – the only one you'll ever have to the day you die – one body to do you forever. What will you do to ensure that you will be able to live well in this body for as many years as you have?

As the patient considers this, I reflect on the lack of common sense of someone who smokes, drinks to excess, eats the wrong foods and more than necessary, fails to get adequate sleep or exercise, drives too fast etc. Common sense? One would think. But there are two levels of common sense.

LEVELS OF COMMON SENSE

Common sense is more like two levels of one overall concept. The first level is *rational or logical common sense*. This relies on what you understand from the information you have gathered. And you have gathered a lot of information as you have developed as a human being, often simply from living in the world. The most important part of what you understand from all of this isn't what you know already, but what you don't know yet, and being able to recognize this fact and do something about it.

You use this kind of common sense all the time. If you have some rational piece of information about your health – like smoking is not good for my health – you have a choice of acting upon it or not. If you apply your rational common sense, logic dictates that the only prudent course of action is to quit smoking. Whoa – you say. It's not that simple. Actually, it is that simple and I'll help you to come to that decision, too.

The second level of common sense is the basic self or the body's own common sense. This relies on what you know at a deep level. Some might even consider this to be a feeling.

It's related to the concept of intuition, but it's not exactly the same thing. For example, you've just read about a new approach to treating arthritis on an Internet web site. You're tempted to jump right in and purchase that seemingly expensive bottle of tablets. It's a breakthrough! At least, that's what the web site says. In any case, your current medications don't seem to be helping as much as you'd like, and you've noticed some unpleasant side effects that can probably be attributed to them. But something tells you that it's too good to be true.

> *Everybody gets so much information all day long that they lose their common sense.* ~ Gertrude Stein

After all, if this treatment is really as good as they say, then why doesn't everyone use it. Why hasn't your doctor recommended it? Why isn't it the only one? Oh, that's probably because it's an alternative approach and everyone knows that doctors are all sceptical of alternative medicine, right? What's wrong with this way of thinking?

There are two common sense errors here. The first one you have heard countless times before: if you have a feeling that something is too good to be true, it probably is. You have no specialized knowledge about this, but you have a feeling. Second, common sense would tell you that sweeping generalizations like "all doctors are sceptical of alternative medicine" isn't true either. Perhaps some are, but making this kind of generalization fails to respect your own intellect. You are electing to create a narrative to validate a decision you have already made. Common sense always respects your intellect.

Even more important when it comes to this less rational type of common sense, your body actually senses things. There is even a firm foundation in human physiology to support this. If you need a more concrete, scientific explanation, then you've come to the right place. The body's fight or flight response is a chemical response that is often triggered by nothing more than sensing something. You sense danger. Your heart begins to pound. Your mouth starts to feel dry. You're on the edge of your seat, ready to flee or to fight. This is your body common sense. We'll take a more in-depth look at the scientific basis in Chapter Four.

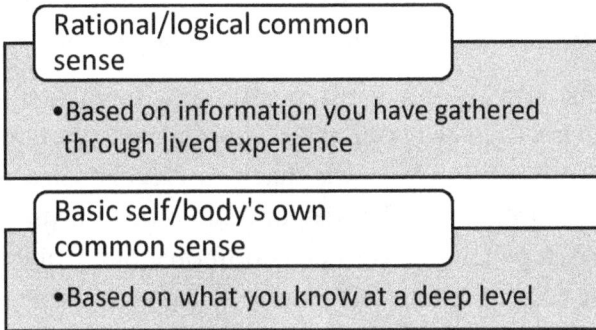

Rational/logical common sense
- Based on information you have gathered through lived experience

Basic self/body's own common sense
- Based on what you know at a deep level

The bottom line is that your own common sense isn't really available to you if you don't trust yourself. It's a simple equation:

Intellect + intuition = good use of common sense

You understand things intellectually, and you also sense things. But if you don't listen to both your intellect and your intuition, you'll continue to be like so many people in the world today: walking around not knowing how you're going to get through life. Your intuition is always with you, speaking to you even if you aren't listening. However, if you never pay attention, at some point it will stop talking.

BEING RESPONSIBLE: THE KEY TO OUR COMMON SENSE

If you go back to the beginning of our story just before this chapter, you can see two different women with two vastly different responses to the situations of their lives. Each one has made a choice to respond in a particular way. They have used their ability to respond. They are largely "response-able" for their current state of affairs. Responsibility is the key to common sense.

Responsibility is often misconstrued with burden. It's no more a burden than are your children – but they certainly are a parent's responsibility. It means that you can choose a response and to be accountable for that response. In other words, you may not be able to change external conditions that come at you throughout your life, but you certainly do have control over how you respond to them – it's your responsibility. And life is full of responsibility – try as you might, you can't get away from it.

There's a Zen proverb that is especially telling: "After the ecstasy, the laundry." Even when you have reached what you consider to be the most exalted status in your life, you are still ultimately responsible for whatever happens after that – and much of it will be mundane.

Accepting responsibility as a part of your life, or taking responsibility if you like, means the ultimate control over your own life. If you take responsibility for your own decisions, then you are, indeed, in control. On the other hand, if you choose to give it away, you lose control. How might you be giving away your responsibility?

One way that's becoming all too familiar to us in modern society is the victim mentality. If you choose to see yourself as a victim in the events of your past, for example, you place the responsibility, and the blame, for your current situation somewhere outside yourself. By doing so you give up any control you might otherwise have had to change the circumstances of your current life. So, maybe you didn't cause your own cancer, but by looking for an external place to hold responsible (e.g. your next-door neighbour's use of lawn chemicals), you abdicate your responsibility to do something about your situation in the present moment. Common sense tells you that you can't change the past – but by focusing on the past, you never get over it. Even Oprah Winfrey has something to say about this. She's been quoted as saying, "My philosophy is that not only are you responsible for your life but doing the best at this moment puts you in the best place for the next moment." (Much more about this in Chapter 11.)

FINDING BALANCE

If responsibility is the key, balance is the mechanism by which you apply your own common sense. This is a two-way situation: If you choose a balanced approach, you are applying common sense; also, if you use common sense, you live a well-balanced life.

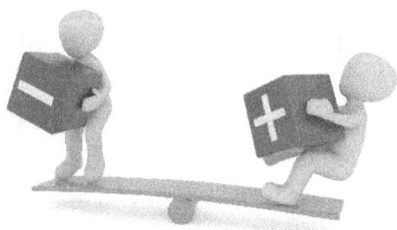

American psychologist, the late Paul Pearsall, author of *The Pleasure Principle* (an original Freudian concept suggesting that people generally seek pleasure and avoid pain) has written about the Hawaiian concept of *pono* – balance. It's his view, and the view of countless others including Buddhist sages, that a middle way that finds the natural balance in all things is the most effective way to achieve health and contentment in life. But imbalance is so common in daily life that we've almost come to see it as normal.

Here are some common imbalances that cause innumerable health problems:

- overwork
- excess working out
- lack of physical activity
- overeating
- under-eating

All the above imbalances cause illness. We need to move away from the philosophy if some is good, then more is better. This just isn't so.

So, you might say, I don't do any of those things to excess, but I still suffer from this or that illness. One of the most important truths that you already know, but that you must truly accept, is that people get sick: it's part of the human condition. It's widely believed that accepting certain truths results in inner peace – if you stop fighting against the truth, you can move on. Peace can have incredible healing qualities – it can even cure sometimes. It's useful to remember that while medicine and its practitioners can cure illnesses, it's up to the individual to heal him or herself. Another way of visualizing balance as the mechanism to unlocking common sense is to picture a teeter-totter. Not only does the weight of each side have an impact on its ability to balance, but also how far the load is away from the centre: the farther out the load is, the more imbalanced it becomes.

There are essentially three ways to achieve balance:

1. Reduce the size of one load (to make them equal).
2. Increase the size of one load (to make them equal).
3. Move both loads toward the centre or balance point.

If we perceive the load as an external condition over which we have little control, maintaining balance requires us to behave in ways that are extreme. If we accept responsibility for our own life, then we move to the centre where the movements are less noticeable.

We all have the potential to be in balance. At the same time, we all have what psychologists sometimes call a "shadow" side, although many people (probably most) fail to recognize theirs. And some who do see it, ignore or deny it. This shadow side is an exaggerated projection of the opposite of what we present to the world. For example, if you find that you are overly concerned about working out so that you can keep your body in top shape, your shadow side is probably a fat, lazy couch potato. It lurks there, just below the surface, and your fear of becoming what your shadow side says is your potential keeps you driving yourself into exhaustion. The bigger the couch potato, the more you have to push your exercise routine in order to maintain balance. This results in your imbalanced behaviour that carries with it the risk of harming your mental and physical health. If you recognize and make friends with your shadow side and choose not to behave in a way that would turn you into your shadow, you can move toward achieving a state of balance and thus better health. It's like having a small child who craves attention. The more you ignore him, the more he acts up. If you give him attention when he acts up, it reinforces the behaviour you want to stop. It's common sense!

There is, however, one more important truth about balance and its ability to activate your common sense: there are no quick fixes. Everything takes time. In today's fast-paced society where fast food and drive-through everything are the norm, expectations are high that we can – and must – "fix" whatever is wrong with us quickly. Therefore, there has been a proliferation of supposed quick fixes marketed to us by everyone from drug companies to celebrities via television, magazines and the

Internet. If you recognize that there are no fast ways to achieve this balance and thus good health, you'll apply common sense to evaluating those offers of fast weight loss, cured cancer, relief from arthritis – all designed to take money from the vulnerable and thus gullible.

Staying balanced isn't always easy – and sometimes seems almost impossible. But the bottom line is that the resources you need to do so are already part of you.

THE TRUTH: YOU ALREADY KNOW WHAT TO DO

Within every living organism on this planet is the remarkable ability to heal. But healing doesn't always mean "cure," at least according to how most of us define the two terms. It's interesting to note, though, that the word cure comes from the Latin *cura* which means to care. Traditionally, this kind of cure meant the successful medical treatment of a disease. Healing, on the other hand, has now come to mean the restoration of balance of mind, body and spirit. You can be cured of a disease in medical terms, yet not be healed. It is also possible to be healed while a disease is still present or even when death is imminent.

If you look back at how we defined health earlier in this chapter, you'll see that these two concepts aren't the same thing. But the bottom line is that you are seeking to be healed from a variety of factors that interfere with your attainment of ideal health – for you. This concept may require some considerable change in your way of thinking – but it's key to your ability to use common sense in your health decisions.

APPLYING THE COMMON SENSE APPROACH TO LIFE AND HEALTH

A common sense approach to your health is simple. It requires the following three things of you:

1. Knowing yourself and your multi-dimensional personality better;

2. Recognizing that your attitude affects how you see your health and health care; and

3. Embracing an action orientation toward a goal of balance.

This means that every time you're faced with a decision about your health, or you have to re-evaluate a current approach based on new external conditions or new information, you don't jump in headfirst without evaluating how this will affect the balance of your life.

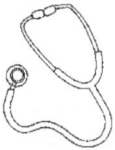

KEYS TO THE COMMON SENSE APPROACH

☑ Everyone, including you, possesses common sense.

☑ "Health" is an individual thing; your optimum health is different from others' optimum health.

☑ Part of using common sense is accepting certain truths; one of the most important is the fact that you won't live forever. Life is terminal.

☑ Intellect plus intuition equals good use of common sense.

☑ The key to using the common sense approach to your life and health is taking responsibility; this is the ultimate control.

☑ Balance is the mechanism by which you apply common sense.

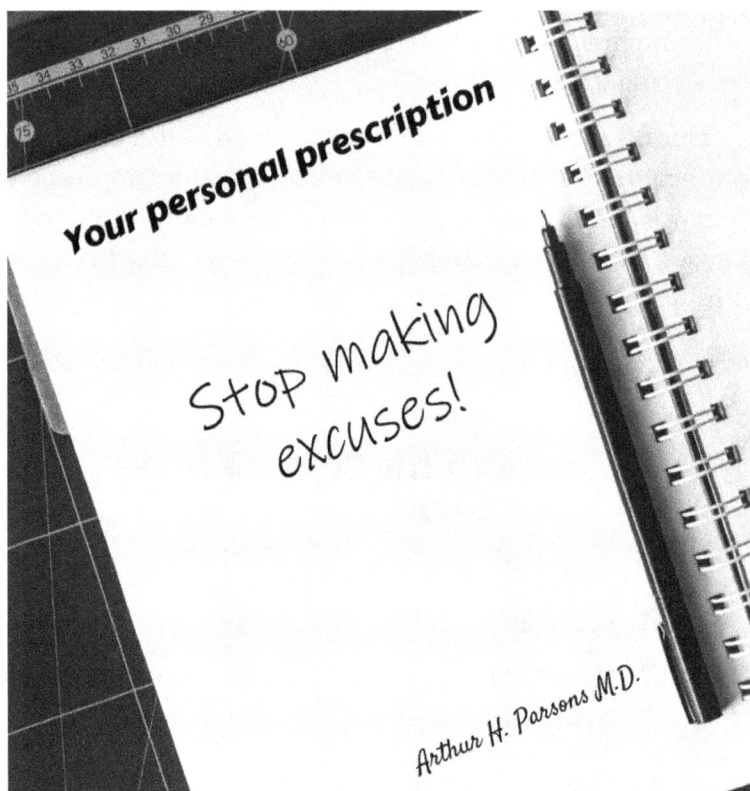

Your personal prescription

Stop making excuses!

Arthur H. Parsons M.D.

CHAPTER TWO

THE BELIEF BACKLASH

"There are things I can't force. I must adjust. There are times when the greatest change needed is a change of my viewpoint." ~
C.M. Ward

IF YOU'RE EVEN A LITTLE BIT INTERESTED in the self-help movement, you can't help but have noticed how many books and positive-thinking gurus continue to promote the concept that your beliefs hold the key to the manifestation of your dreams – in other words, if you think positively, and change your beliefs to positive ones, life will unfold as you desire. What they often fail to address, however, is what I call the *belief backlash*. Developing a positive belief system without addressing what lies beneath your current beliefs – why you hold certain beliefs – can have a kind of backlash effect. While it seems that a positive belief system can't be anything but good for you, it isn't enough.

How many truisms do you personally hold about your health? You know the ones. Things like these: If you sit on a cold surface, you'll develop hemorrhoids or a bladder infection. If you sleep in a draft or go out without sufficiently warm clothing, you'll develop a cold.

25

And you can probably think up many more such "truisms" that have been passed down to you from family members, or even foisted on you by well-meaning, but mistaken friends. The truth is that many people project their beliefs onto others regularly. It's important for them to compel you to believe in the same things the same way that they do, so that their own belief can be reinforced. This is how culture develops.

Take a moment to think about your own health-related beliefs then consider how many times you've been correct. In other words, you got a chill last year, then you came down with a cold. Thus, you conclude that getting a chill caused your cold, so your belief holds true, and you're sticking to it. You come to this conclusion despite all scientific explanations indicating quite clearly that you need to contract a cold virus to get a cold. You interpret your perceptions through your core beliefs.

But do you really *know* these things? Truly know them? There's a world of difference between what you believe and what you truly know to be true.

Your body is the outward manifestation of your mind and your beliefs. If you think of your body as a kind of amazing computer, then it's clear that we have a phenomenal potential to achieve our own personal level of good health. But like any other computer, it is nothing *but* potential if we don't have the appropriate software. ***Our beliefs are our personal software.***

Another way you may like to think about this is the way practitioners of Traditional Chinese Medicine do. Our body is less a technological marvel, than it is a garden, to be nurtured and cared for. But a beautiful garden doesn't just exist on its own. Although the sunlight and the water may be provided by nature, a cultivated garden also needs soil amendments on a regular basis. And it is the gardener who provides those amendments. Your beliefs are the amendments. If they change from time to time, the results will vary.

FIGURING OUT WHAT A BELIEF REALLY IS

It's likely you've never really stopped to consider what a belief really is. If you're going to figure out how to use your own beliefs to the best advantage of your health and life, then you need to understand exactly what it is you may have to work on.

Webster's dictionary defines a belief as "probable knowledge." Note carefully that it doesn't indicate that belief and knowledge are the same thing, only that a belief is *probable* knowledge. It might be knowledge; but it might not be. It also suggests that a belief is "an acceptance of something as true or actual."

> **A belief is something you accept to be true regardless of its provenance.**

Something that you believe and something that is objectively true are not necessarily the same thing. In spite of what you might think when you consider your own beliefs, especially about your health, what's lacking in them is any degree of certainty. *Beliefs are not facts* (no matter what we may be seeing in the media these days). As I said before, you may believe that if you get chilled you will develop a cold, even though you are intellectually aware that you need to contract a cold virus to develop a cold. Getting chilled might, however, actually depress your immune system thus allowing the virus to take hold and cause you to develop a cold. Facts applied to your belief system can result in a good dose of common sense.

We often say to other people, and more importantly to ourselves, that we *know* this, or we *know* that. The truth is that what we are usually talking about is what we *believe*. Sometimes it's nothing more than an opinion. We often lack enough factual information to be able to internalize the belief into a true, heartfelt "knowing." If you are really honest with yourself, you'll soon recognize those beliefs you hold to be true about yourself and your health are really only "probable knowledge" rather than real "knowings."

Here's a summary of the difference between what you *believe* and what you *know*.

What You Believe	What You Know
• Your beliefs are handed to you from external sources. • There is some doubt, however small, attached to your beliefs. • Believing in something is a mental exercise. • Believing something can restrict you. • Beliefs are changeable depending upon the acquisition of new information.	• What you know to be true comes from within yourself. • There is no doubt attached thus what you know is reliable. • What you know is in the physical domain. • What you know can empower you. • If you truly know something, that knowing can't be changed by new information.

Every once in a while, what you believe comes face to face with what you truly know to be true. This is especially true when it comes to health and illness. When a *knowing* faces a *belief*, the knowing always triumphs. For example, you may have begun to believe that as long as you are fit (i.e. in good physical condition

28

as defined by some source), your obesity doesn't matter. This belief was likely handed to you by some media "influencer" (or at least from someone outside yourself), and you probably harbour some doubt about the veracity of this belief, especially since you know not everyone agrees with this. It's a mental exercise that doesn't require you to take any other action. So,

> *The trouble with the world is not that people know too little, but that they know so many things that ain't so.* ~ Mark Twain

you believe it, but do you really *know* that your obesity doesn't matter if you consider yourself to be fit? No, you don't. Since you must defend this stance, it is merely what you believe, not what you know. If you knew it, there would be no doubt, and you would feel empowered.

Now that you recognize the difference between what you believe and what you truly know, we'll take a closer look at where these beliefs come from and what you may be able to do about the ones that are interfering with your ability to access your common sense.

THE PROVENANCE OF WHAT YOU BELIEVE AND WHAT YOU KNOW

Our thoughts are rehearsal sessions for the beliefs we carry. Consider a typical day.

When you arise in the morning, you take a shower. Instead of just being in the shower while the water flows over you, enjoying that moment for what it is, you're concentrating on a meeting you have later in the day. The meeting is with someone you don't know well, but you've heard some rumours about his bad temper and his negative attitude toward your project. You begin to dwell on these rumours. Before you know it, you begin to believe that these rumours represent the nature of the man, so you plan your approach based on this. You have no facts to support this belief; no personal observations for example, but that doesn't matter. Then you have breakfast. While drinking your coffee, you listen to the news on the radio. You hear a report about a suspected outbreak of a new disease in your region which many sufferers believe is the result of being exposed to fluorescent light. You listen to the litany of symptoms which include fatigue and itchy skin. You are tired and sometimes find yourself scratching. You have fluorescent lights in your office. Despite medical studies to the contrary, you begin to believe that such exposure is damaging your health. That's your story and you're sticking to it.

Many of the rationalizations we use to defend our beliefs and excuse our behaviour are, in fact, lies. But, generally speaking, the only person who will be directly hurt by your lies is you. However, if for example, you are a so-called "anti-vaxxer", someone who does not believe in vaccinations for whatever reason despite all the science supporting them, whenever you convince others to follow your lead, you have put more than just yourself and your family at risk, since vaccination is more a public health issue than a personal health one.

The problem with the above story is that it really isn't so fictitious. It is played out in many people's lives day after day. We begin to think about something and the more we think about it and put various disparate thoughts together, the easier it is for us to believe almost anything. And damn the truth. These kinds of negative thoughts and subsequent belief systems are a powerful part of the belief backlash. But we continue to hold on to these negative beliefs that interfere with the quality of our lives.

Writer and creativity guru, Julia Cameron, believes that we maintain our negative beliefs because we feel safer with them than without them.

In her book *The Artist's Way*, she says, "We may not be happy, at least we know what we are – unhappy." She applies this to the concept of creativity where negative beliefs may prevent us from taking risks. Isn't it just possible that any negative beliefs you have about your own health may also be a safe haven for you?

For example, if you were in perfect health, wouldn't people expect more from you? Wouldn't you expect yourself to be more productive, more energetic, more effective? This can sometimes be a frightening or worrisome prospect. Even if this doesn't faze you, you're probably wondering how it is you came to hold such beliefs that have a negative impact on your health and life.

We are brought up to live by other people's should's, ought-to's, have-to's and must-do's. This external input has a powerful effect on our

Human behavior flows from three main sources: desire, emotion, and knowledge. ~ Plato

thought processes resulting in each of us developing our own set of beliefs that get us through our days. These beliefs explain and rationalize a wide variety of behaviour.

If you take a more social science approach to determining the genesis of your beliefs, you might consider the three ways we acquire our beliefs, and ultimately what we believe we know.

- BY INTUITION: We simply feel that something is a particular way. Subconscious thoughts and feelings that are a result of our exposure to people and ideas contribute to this, but in the end, you can't really put your finger on where the belief came from other than you just "know" it or so you say.

- BY TENACITY: This means hanging on to an idea because it's always been that way. You tenaciously hold on to beliefs that come from your youth for example, not daring to give them up.

- BY AUTHORITY: This is one of the most common ways we develop our beliefs – as a result of what someone who appears to us to know more than we do tells us. These people who seem to be authorities on certain subjects are often only expounding on their own beliefs – and this can apply to doctors and other experts as well. These are also people like parents, clergy, people we like, television personalities, internet personalities etc. Although there may be some value in looking to authority figures for knowledge, any information they provide to form the basis for your belief system has to be taken a step further before you can truly say you know something.

- DIRECT EXPERIENCE: Real knowing comes from action and experience. You need to act on some of the information and ideas handed to you so that you can really internalize them and relinquish the doubt that is associated with so many of our beliefs. The problem with these beliefs is that *we don't attract into our lives what we want, but things that confirm what we believe.*

DIFFERENT KINDS OF BELIEFS

All beliefs are not created equal. We hold different kinds of beliefs, all of which can have different effects on our thought processes, and consequently the decisions that we make that affect our behaviour.

Let's start by examining the broadest category: your *global beliefs*. These beliefs are generalizations – and you know how much trouble generalizations can get you into. The problem is that we often hold global beliefs about which we are almost completely unaware. Consider your own generalizations that relate to your physical, mental and spiritual health.

- Do you hold any global beliefs about what life is like? For example, do you ever say things like: Life is hard. Life is complicated. Life is boring. Life is to be lived to the fullest. As you can see, these are almost like philosophies for living. If you hold any of these, or other similar global beliefs about life and you can identify them, you are starting to uncover your own core beliefs that affect the decisions you make without you even being aware.

- Do you hold any global beliefs about physical health in general or *your* physical health in particular? For example, do you ever say (even to yourself) things like: Sickness just happens; no one has any control over it. Sickness is a weakness. People always cause their own sickness. Again, these kinds of all-encompassing beliefs about health are certain to have insidious effects on your decisions about what and how you will care for your physical self.

- Do you have any global beliefs about your mental health? For example, do you ever say (even to yourself) things like: I'm just a depressed person. I will always be unstable. I'm disorganized. These global beliefs about your mental self have an impact on all other health-related decisions that you will make in your life.

The second category of beliefs is falls under the rubric of **rules**. The trouble with these beliefs is that they often seem so logical. "If this... then that." These rules are those beliefs you hold which tell you that if one set of circumstances occurs, then another one will follow. People hold onto all kinds of rules about their health.

Think hard about what you believe to be circumstances that affect your health. Do you believe any of the following?

- If you sit on cold concrete, you'll get a bladder infection.
- If you sit on cold ground, you'll get hemorrhoids.
- If you have cancer and they operate on you, it will seed the cancer.
- If you sleep in a draft, you'll get a cold.
- If you... well, you get the picture.

You can probably think up your own set of rules (beliefs) that you have developed through your life. None of these actually represents real health facts. But people continue to believe them, and these beliefs interfere with both the acquisition of the truth and the knowledge about what to do about your individual situation.

The key to figuring out why and how your own beliefs are causing you problems is first examining your own beliefs, then determining where your beliefs come into conflict. For example, if you hold certain global beliefs or rules about your health, then you are confronted with the

If you don't change your beliefs, your life will be like this forever. Is that good news? ~ W. Somerset Maugham

facts from someone like your doctor, the ensuing conflict will have negative effects on your relationship with your doctor and on your health. If you are diagnosed with cancer and your doctor recommends surgery to remove the tumor, if you believe that this will "seed" the tumor, you will face a very difficult decision about your treatment options. Indeed, *your belief may even rob you of all options* However, not all beliefs are bad.

There are two very valuable core beliefs that, if you adopt them as part of your personal global belief system and truly take them to heart, may enable you to make good decisions about your health – in fact, they are the first steps toward empowering your common sense. They are as follows:

1. **The past doesn't equal the future**. In other words, your past experiences are just that – in the past. They do not have to dictate what will happen in the future. Things can change, and if you remain open to the possibility of change, you can evolve.

2. **There is always a way if you are committed.** This is a terrific belief to hold that will help you to be open to new ideas and that will propel you toward action.

The past doesn't equal the future.	There is always a way if you are committed.

COMMON SENSICAL OR FOOLISH?

Canadian psychologist Dr. James Alcock, author of the 2018 book *Belief: What it Means to Believe and Why Our Convictions Are So Compelling*, says, "While we generally trust our beliefs and they usually serve us well, they can be very vulnerable to error and distortion." It is these errors and distortions that fool us, and make no mistake, we are all fooled from time to time. It only really becomes a problem when we continually allow ourselves to be fooled by both outside influences as well as our own ill-founded beliefs.

Being fooled is, in effect, the opposite of acting with common sense. There are essentially two ways you can be fooled.

The first is by believing things that are not so. In other words, if you continue to believe and act on things that have no basis in fact, that are not so, then you are not tapping into your own common sense – you are allowing yourself to be fooled.

The second way that you can be fooled is by not believing in things that are actually facts. Sometimes, deep within you, you know certain things to be true, but you refuse to believe them anyway. For example, if you're unhappy with your weight, and it's causing you health-related problems (as weight issues will do), and deep inside you know and understand the calories-in-calories-out concept, but you continue to believe that you're doomed to be fat because everyone in your family is fat (even though you have observed that they take in far more calories than your slimmer friends), or you search for opinions that the calorie-in-calorie-out approach isn't true, then you are failing yourself. Again, you are failing to employ your own common sense.

Why, then, do we continue to fool ourselves? It all comes back to action. If we were to employ our common sense in most situations, we would be forced to take a different course of action and, most often, we would be forced to take responsibility for our own health and life outcomes. You have to do something different. That can be a very intimidating prospect. However, if you don't apply common sense on a regular basis, you must face the outcomes of not doing so, and those outcomes are usually negative in the long run.

THE EFFECTS OF YOUR BELIEFS

Before your knowledge about your beliefs can be truly useful to you, you need to understand what effects these beliefs – both good and bad – can have on you and your health.

We do not attract into our lives what we want; rather we attract the things that confirm what we believe we are. This is not an airy-fairy, new age solecism: your focus does, indeed, determine what you see. Remember what happens when you decide on a new make and model of car to buy? Before you even buy it, you begin to conclude that this car is far more common than you thought. You begin to see them everywhere, even though your common sense tells you that there are no more of these vehicles around this week than there were last week before you did the research and decided to buy one. The only thing that has changed is your focus. It is the same thing when it comes to your health. Your body and its health status are the outward manifestation of your mind *and your beliefs*. This outward manifestation can include your overall appearance, your facial expression, your body language, how you move etc. and as we will discuss later in the book, even your cellular function.

Beliefs can also create victims. If you believe you are ...too short ...too fat ...stupid ... disorganized ...lethargic ... etc. you become a victim of that belief. Victimization is close to lethal for good health. It is almost impossible for you to take responsibility for your own well-being if you believe that you are a victim of some external force over which you have little or no control – whether it's bad genes or an overbearing mother – you will have compromised your belief system and you will almost certainly make decisions that are not congruent with good health.

The bottom line is that everything we think about and come to believe, we project into the world with powerful effects, many of which we cannot predict. There is even some scientific evidence to support the notion that those projections can affect others – even at a distance – and can affect your own cells. (I'll examine this scientific approach in more detail in Chapter Four.)

CAN YOU CHANGE YOUR BELIEFS?

If large companies can mount marketing campaigns to effectively change what you believe about your consumer needs compelling you take action to buy their product, surely you can mount your own internal marketing campaign to change your beliefs that are causing the quality of your life to be less than it could be. So, that's exactly what you're going to do – market new beliefs to yourself. How do you do that?

Have you ever had your evening meal interrupted by a telemarketer or pollster wanting to ask you questions about the products you buy? Just as companies that want to sell you products ask questions to figure out your buying habits and what you think of their products, you need to begin by identifying what unhealthy beliefs you hold, then figure out which one(s) you will tackle. Just as a marketer focuses on one consumer need at a time for maximum effectiveness, you can't expect to deal with a host of dubious beliefs all at once. You'll need to go through the process a number of times.

Once you identify the belief that is interfering with your health and impeding your life's journey, you need to consider all of the negative consequences you have associated it with. Just as a company selling antibacterial wipes will provide you with a litany of the problems that can occur without their product so that you will want to move away from those negative images, you will also need to find that big stick within your own belief. That big stick needs to encompass all of the pain that you have ever associated with that belief – all of the negative consequences that have resulted from it. You need to intercept that pattern of behaviour.

Once you have felt the pain associated with that belief, create a slogan that obliterates the belief and that makes you feel powerful. At this point it doesn't even have to be completely accurate. This slogan is a new, empowering belief that will move you toward action.

Now, just like the marketer with the new wipes will provide you with testimonials of happy people and all of the pleasure that they have associated with that product, you need to link massive pleasure with the new belief. This is the carrot toward which you want to move. Think about the positive consequences.

Finally, just like the marketer keeps bombarding you with the message about the new product, you need to continue to bombard yourself with the new belief by rehearsing over and over again how your life will be better and how painful it would be for you to keep your old belief. Now, just the facts...

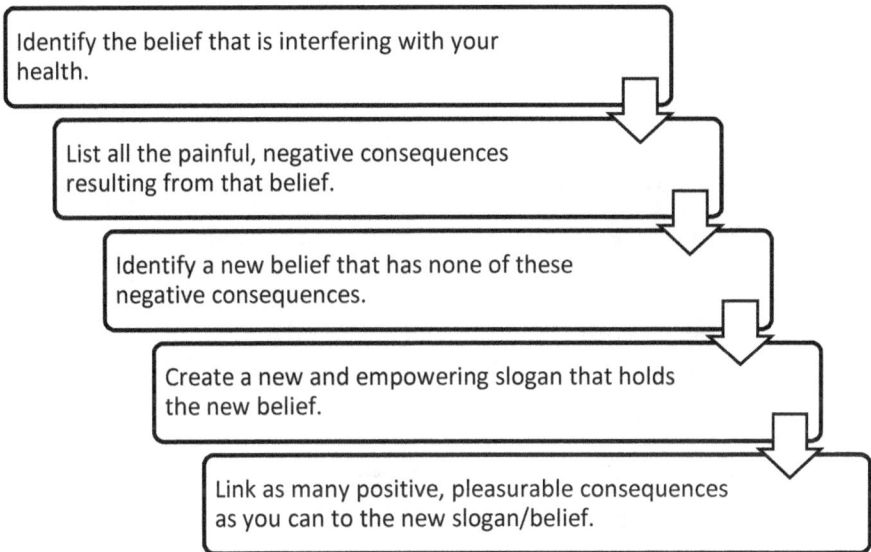

Identify the belief that is interfering with your health.

List all the painful, negative consequences resulting from that belief.

Identify a new belief that has none of these negative consequences.

Create a new and empowering slogan that holds the new belief.

Link as many positive, pleasurable consequences as you can to the new slogan/belief.

...repeat as often as necessary. Just as companies can change your buying behaviour by altering the images in your mind, you can have that same powerful effect on yourself. Why let outside forces manipulate your thinking without having your own input! But, are there any issues with all this positivity? Can you go overboard? I'll answer these questions in the next chapter.

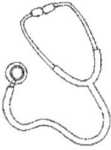

KEYS TO USING YOUR BELIEF SYSTEM

☑ Your beliefs are your personal software and if your software is faulty, the execution of the program will naturally be faulty.

☑ Beliefs are not the same thing as facts.

☑ What you believe is not the same thing as what you know to be true.

☑ Your beliefs may be robbing you of options.

☑ Identify yourself with the observer in you. Simply observe your thoughts, but don't take ownership of them. Don't say, "These are mine," simply because you think them.

☑ One way of working on this detachment from your thoughts, which is so important for health and contentment, is meditation. As a technique it lets you observe your thoughts and let them go.

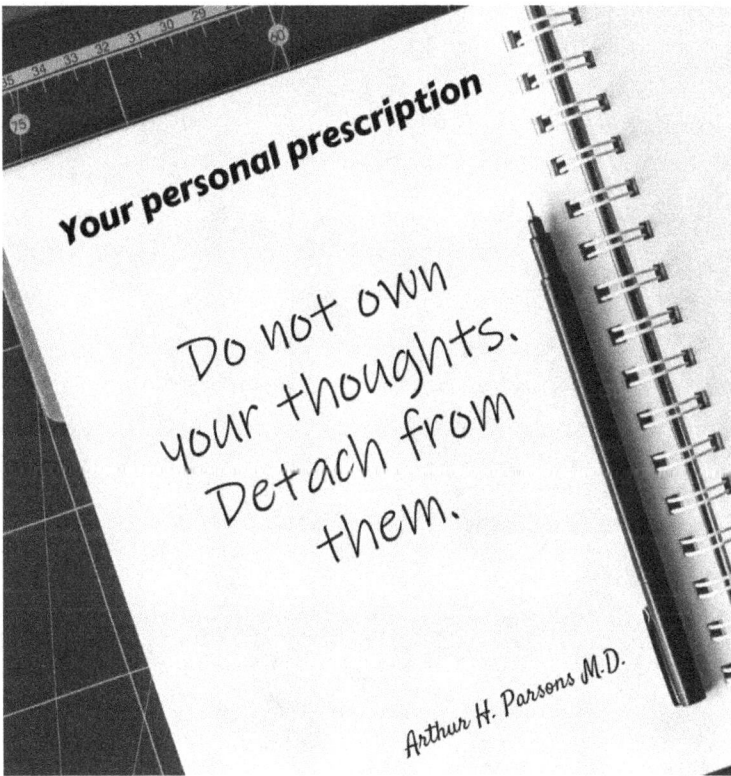

Your personal prescription

Do not own your thoughts. Detach from them.

Arthur H. Parsons M.D.

Parsons

CHAPTER THREE

THE LIMITS OF POSITIVE THINKING

"It's a funny thing about life; if you refuse to accept anything but the best, you very often get it." ~ Somerset Maugham

HOW SICK ARE YOU OF ALL THAT POSITIVE ATTITUDE STUFF that we've been subjected to for the past decade or two? Wouldn't you just like to slap that smiling, toothy grin off that guy on the cover of his book? You know the one: it's the one that tells you if you just think positively all the time, and never let a negative thought enter your head, you'll get everything you ever wanted in life. Maybe you're like many of us who are interested in the relationship between our thinking and its outcomes in our lives and on our health, and you've given it a try. Then, failing to manifest your wildest dreams, you begin to think you're a failure – a negative frame of mind if ever there was one. Or, maybe you know people who are really trying to incorporate this positive thinking into their lives. They are always "great", there is never a problem (only situations), and life is beautiful. These people can be trying, indeed.

The truth is: life is not a complete bowl of cherries; suffering is a part of the human condition. If you were never sad, you'd have a lot of trouble recognizing happiness. It's that very state of heartache that makes us able to savour the deliciousness of the contentment, delight and peace when we are truly in balance.

Pain is certain, suffering is optional. ~ Gautama Buddha

Common sense comes to the rescue. Common sense tells you that no one is happy all the time; it just isn't possible, nor even a state that would be beneficial for your life. There is however, a distinct relationship between your attitude and your health. The notion that a positive spin on your attitude can have positive health benefits may not be news to you: you just may need to look at it differently.

Contrary to what voracious consumers of new age gurus might think, a negative attitude is not the only thing that contributes to illness and you are not responsible for every problem that befalls you. This is a faulty way of considering the notion of taking responsibility for your health and the decisions affecting it. But the relationship between attitude and health is indeed worth considering, and how you respond to those problems that befall you is indeed under your control.

Your attitude, the attitude of those around you and even your doctor's attitude can all have an impact on the health care that you receive and how you respond to it.

EXACTLY WHAT IS AN "ATTITUDE"?

You probably use this word a lot. You discuss your children's attitudes, your boss's attitude, and your family's attitude.

Sometimes you're referring to something on an emotional level, but frequently people mix this up with a more intellectual approach. What, then, are we really talking about?

In Chapter Two we discussed your beliefs. Although there is a close relationship between your beliefs and your attitudes, they are two different things. Here's how we can define attitude:

An attitude is the sum total of the thoughts, feelings and emotional states you attach to any particular issue.

Another way of looking at your attitude is to consider it to be the result of making judgments about the beliefs you hold. Although it is true that you likely have specific attitudes about specific issues, I'm referring to a more general philosophical approach toward your life. In this case you can have only one of three possible overall attitudes: positive, negative or neutral. Overall (but not exclusively), you feel mostly optimistic about your life and your health, or you feel pessimistic, or you feel apathetic.

These emotional states (as opposed to intellectual beliefs) paint your life and health with a particular colour, and you see issues relating to life and health as if through a pair of glasses tinted in a particular direction. It might occur to you that a neutral attitude, making you generally apathetic toward your life might provide you with the clearest view. However, that so-called clear view, that results in a kind of fatalistic approach to your life, is often as problematic as a pessimistic approach.

Your attitude then, is…

- a state of being,

- your outlook on your life,

- the viewpoint from which you see your world,

- the approach you take to decisions about your life and health, and

- the demeanour you exhibit to others.

Your attitude is not just one of these things; rather it is all of them. If your intellectual beliefs and the events outside of yourself are the water and wind that act upon the ship of your life, then your attitude is the way you set your sail. The set of your sail is completely under your control. As American tennis player & activist Judith M. Knowlton once said, "I discovered I always have choices and sometimes it's only a choice of attitude."

WHERE OUR ATTITUDES COME FROM

You weren't born with your attitudes. There doesn't seem to be any evidence to support a conviction that our attitudes are in any way genetic. Where did your attitudes come from, then? The attitudes that you carry around with you every day – and that you're more than willing to share with others in the form of your opinions, actions and general demeanour – are the sum product of a number of factors. In fact, your attitudes are a bit like a big stew. There are many ingredients all of which are mixed together for a while and left to simmer.

Let's start with the influencing factor that has probably already come to your mind: your attitudes are largely influenced by your family circumstances. The family structure, how it functions and interacts and the values that your family lives by all play a part in how you develop your way of thinking about particular subjects, and your overall view of life. If you have a family that was supportive of you as a child and looked favourably upon your endeavours, this may play a part in your development of a positive attitude. Although it certainly isn't the only influence. Nor can you truly blame your family for your negative approach to life, since some people are able to use their negative family attitudes to develop opposite, positive ones as a reaction to all the negativity.

Another important general set of factors that has already influenced your attitudes is the culture/race/creed set. Your culture, and its inherent beliefs and values will influence your attitudes. It is possible that the way you think about things is in line with those cultural influences, but it might be the case that your attitudes have developed in direct reaction to them resulting in opposite attitudes. It's just as likely that the influence could be more moderate. The same is true of your religion and social/economic background. When it comes to the influence of race, your attitudes are most likely affected by how you perceive yourself and your racial group to be viewed by society, rather than there being any specific attitudes generally held by people of any given race. For example, if as a child, people reacted to your racial characteristics negatively, this will have an effect on how you view any number of issues as you grow up.

Another factor in the development of how you see the world is your educational background. This includes the kind of education and the level you have achieved. But, remember, education goes beyond the classroom. What you have learned from your travels around the world, for example, may cause you to see things differently. If you have a grade school education, the way you see your world will be different (not worse or better – just different) than the way a person with a medical degree will view it. On the other hand, two people who possess doctoral degrees – one in economics and one in Romance literature – both have the same level of education but may have drastically differing attitudes toward any number of issues.

Twenty-first century life has brought with it another, increasingly and singularly potent influence on attitudes – social media and the internet. There is mounting evidence that attitudes displayed toward everything from political machinations to disease treatments are massively affected by the social media habits of individuals. Who you follow, how much you interact, why you seek out information – these are some of the factors that affect the extent to which your personal attitudes have been manipulated by the internet. The fact that we now refer to a whole set of individuals as "social media influencers" only begins to tell the story. (More about this in Chapter Six.)

Finally, and probably the only one that may have some basis in genetics, is the issue of personal characteristics. This means that certain physical characteristics that you possess, whether it's a large nose or beautiful blonde hair, and how you perceive these things are viewed by the world will influence you. Additionally, if you have been healthy all your life, you may have different attitudes toward the healthcare system, for example, than someone who has been chronically ill and often in the hospital since childhood. You might be asking, but what about life experience in general? Doesn't that count for something? Of course. But life experience is usually related to one of the above characteristics.

> *It's not what happens to you, but how you react to it that matters.* ~ Epictetus

Just as you can adjust the sails of a boat depending on the wind and water conditions, so too can you adjust and change your attitudes to afford you smooth sailing on the seas of life. Some people will adjust the sails only if they are forced to do so by external conditions; however, canny people who are able to tap into their common sense will make small and frequent adjustments to stay on course. This obviates the need for those major adjustments.

Before we move away from what gave you your attitudes, consider again that attitudes can generally be divided into positive, negative or neutral. Consider this differentiation as you examine your list of influences to determine for yourself how your own attitudes fit into these categories. Then consider unplugging yourself from thoughts and events that have a negative authority over you.

THOUGHTS & JUDGMENTS & EXPECTATIONS

Everything is thought. All relationships are thought. The past is thought. Your experience is thought. Your expectations for the future are thought. Since you can control your thoughts, you can, therefore, do anything at all that you want with them. And it's worth considering that many of the thoughts we have aren't accurate anyway.

Think about that power for a minute. Think about your relationships, for example. What does a relationship look like? Can you draw a picture of your relationship with your spouse? Your son? If you're angry with your son for not living up to your expectations, can you see those expectations floating there in your relationship? Can anyone else see them or feel them or touch them? Or are they your thoughts and only your thoughts? What would happen if you changed your thoughts? If you began to consider a different way of thinking about your son's behaviour, it's possible that your relationship would change – it has to. Change your thought processes and your emotional attachments to those thoughts, and you change your life.

More than a decade ago, pop-psychology guru, the late Dr. Wayne Dyer, wrote a popular book titled Change Your Thoughts; Change Your Life, and since then, many people have elaborated on this concept. However, before any of the modern-day gurus even considered this possibility, ancient philosophers had already suggested this as a way forward:

- Roman emperor and philosopher Marcus Aurelius is believed to have said, "The happiness of your life depends on the quality of your thoughts."

- The Buddha is quoted as having said, "The mind is everything – what you think, you become."

It isn't a new idea. But it is one that many people forget. Before you actually take any action in your life, there is a thought that precedes it.

It seems, then, that common sense would tell you that pain and suffering in your emotional life are simply the difference between what is and what you want it to be. What follows logically is that if you change what you want, the pain and suffering will diminish.

"As you think, so shall you be." Lots of people have said that, or something very similar. In fact, there's a plethora of pop-psychology and new age books on this very subject. If you've spent any time reading this material or listening to the gurus, you probably already know that the mantra is "think your way to health and happiness." Whereas there are many good ideas and philosophies in all of this material, the idea of just using your thought processes to manifest all manner of conditions in your life (health, wealth) seems to run contrary to your common sense. You may have a gut reaction that it can't be that simple. And you're right.

Although changing your way of looking at something – your paradigm – causes a shift in your psyche, it takes more than simply thinking about it. It also takes acting upon that new way of thinking. For example, you can't think yourself into good health if you don't change your behaviour to support those thoughts. This brings us to the concept of affirmations.

WHEN YOU WISH UPON A ... YOU KNOW THE REST

An affirmation is usually defined as a statement about what you desire in your life made in such a way that it sounds like you have already accomplished it. Or, in other words, a statement about the future, made in the present, as if it had already happened in the past. Here are some examples:

- If you are struggling with weight loss, you are supposed to say to yourself something like, "It is wonderful now that I have lost weight, and am feeling healthy."

- If you are depressed, you are supposed to say to yourself something like, "I am content with my life and moving toward my goals."

- If you want to quit smoking, you are supposed to say to yourself something like, "I am a non-smoker. I feel comfortable and healthy."

And you're supposed to repeat these statements to yourself on a daily basis.

The idea that affirmations can work is based on the belief that we attract into our lives what we think about. For example, if all you can think about is how unhealthy you feel, then it's going to be very difficult for you to do anything about your unhealthy behaviour until you start to consider the possibility of health. This is where affirmations come in, and they do have their place. But they are not without their problems.

Common sense – your own intellect coupled with your intuitive take on this – might be telling you that if you're 50 pounds overweight, just telling yourself that you're not isn't going to change anything if your self-image is of a fat person. An affirmation that is contrary to what you believe intellectually will not be effective and isn't really honest. We do not attract into our lives what we wish for and want, rather we attract confirmations of what we believe at our core we are. Thus, there is a difference between a wish and an affirmation. Just trying to think yourself thin is completely nonsensical without considering the behaviour changes that will have to be accomplished before even an ounce of weight comes off.

Most people's so-called positive thinking is wishing, not believing. This is really important – most people's so-called positive thinking is wishing, not believing. And if this is true for you, then using affirmations will not give you the same effects as it will for people who are able to change their core beliefs about what and who they are. If you can come to believe that you are not really a fat person, just a normal weight person who has accumulated too much excess weight, then focusing your thoughts on healthy eating and the benefits of exercise just might help you to alter your unhealthy behaviour, then you'll see results.

Adopting the right attitude can convert a negative stress into a positive one. ~ Hans Selye

---

EXCUSE ME, YOUR ATTITUDES ARE SHOWING

As much as you might think that you are keeping your attitudes to yourself, they show in almost everything you do. They're like your signature on every action you take. And this is true whether the actions you take are deliberate, planned approaches, or impulsive, acting-before-thinking conduct.

Let's look first at your impulsive, seat-of-the-pants kind of behaviour. We're all subject to it from time to time, while a few have taken impulsivity on as a way of life. This is the kind of behaviour that shows your attitudes in their most raw form. This means that if you act impetuously, without clear forethought, whatever attitudes you might hold about something will be the guiding force of your action. You will have had little time to examine the potential outcomes of what you are saying or doing. This does not always have positive results, especially if your attitudes are not positive toward the matter.

On the other hand, you may think that if you avoid such capricious action, your attitudes will stay hidden and you can act in any way that suits your fancy. The problem is that you can't hide from your attitudes. They will naturally creep into whatever you do, regardless of how deliberate and planned it might be. It's a bit like telling a newspaper reporter something "off the record." While that reporter may, in fact, not use your information directly, it will doubtless colour any further interviews he or she does, and subsequently have an impact on what is eventually reported. However, unlike the off-the-record comment over which you have total control, unless you have taken the time to develop and control your attitudes toward any number of issues, you won't have the luxury of simply not using them.

The bottom line in all of this…

> **…action that grows naturally from your self-awareness is much more powerful than any impulsive action you might take…**

If you get to know yourself, and are conscious of the attitudes you hold, your action will be genuine, and it will have more profound and authentic results. You need to ensure that you are conscious of both your attitudes and the actions in your life that they spawn.

FALSE FACES: HOW POSITIVITY CAN HURT

Common sense and even the Buddha tell us that it isn't possible to be positive about everything all the time. On some level, it might seem like a good thing if everyone, everywhere, had a positive approach to everything. If you ignore the suffering that is inherent to human life, refusing to feel the intensity, you will soon lose the ability to feel the intensity of the powerfully positive experiences of your life. Putting a false face of positivity on everything can be harmful to your development as a human being, and ultimately to your health.

As I mentioned earlier, over the past decade or two, an extensive industry has grown up around the concept of positivity. There are books, seminars, podcasts, videos, experts, gurus – and everything that goes along with propping up any industry. All of this positivity has become just a bit hard to take for anyone with a shred of common sense.

In 2012, British journalist Oliver Burkeman published The Antidote: Happiness for People Who Can't Stand Positive Thinking, a book intended to provide, as the title suggests, an antidote to the positivity foisted on the public by this multi-billion-dollar industry. In it he suggests that one of the things that makes people unhappy, negative if you like, is chasing happiness and positivity – and failing to reach it. It seems that all that grasping toward the positive is making us positively negative. Even a 2016 study by three academics in New York and Hamburg, Germany suggested that although positive thinking can help conditions like depression in the short-term, over the long run it can actually make it worse. Being positive and having a positive attitude, however, are not the same thing. Common sense about a positive attitude toward life means exploring both sides of something and finding balance that supports good decisions. Putting a positive spin on everything isn't the same as exploring that point of balance which ultimately gives you a generally positive attitude – it allows you to see both sides of a situation.

For example, if you are faced with a health problem such as a cancer diagnosis, it might seem at first glance to be comforting to be able to put a positive spin on this, as some health and self-help gurus suggest. "This is a good thing. I need this. This might be fun." Huh? Doesn't sound very common sensical does it? The first time you're faced with a chemotherapy session, you'll find that it isn't very much fun at all (although you might need the chemo, you probably don't really think you need the cancer at this point), and your false face will shatter like a mirror struck with a hammer. You'll be left in pieces with a feeling of being betrayed – by yourself. This is not helpful to you.

On the other hand, if you are honest with yourself, and you carry a generally positive approach to life, you'll start by evaluating both sides – the suffering and the joy. You may understand that this is an opportunity for personal growth, as any powerful life experience can be, but you'll also recognize that it will be a difficult and perhaps physically painful situation. Years ago, in a James Bond book, author Ian Fleming said this: "You only live twice: once when you are born and once when you face death." Many people don't pay attention to their lives, but when they face a cancer diagnosis for example, they face death, and sometimes it is only then that they begin to live and make positive changes.

Somewhere between the two extremes of thought – negative and positive – you will come to that balance point. It is that point of balance – which is not apathy – where your common sense kicks in and you are able to use this attitude to help yourself.

YOUR ATTITUDE & YOUR HEALTH CARE

It is probably becoming clear to you that there is a distinct relationship between your attitude and your health. But there is also a connection between your attitude and your health CARE. The kind of health care you receive and how you respond to it are dependent at least in part on the way you see things – because how you see things and the attitude that shows (we have already discussed how your attitude shows) is what people who affect your health care will respond to.

Let's look first at your relationship with your doctor (or other primary healthcare provider) and how your attitude may be having an effect in this area. Take a moment to answer the following questions:

☐ Do you feel comfortable when chatting with your doctor?

☐ Do you feel comfortable while you are waiting for your appointment?

☐ Do you expect to receive good care?

☐ Do you like your doctor?

☐ Do you believe your doctor?

☐ Do you trust your doctor?

☐ Do you follow your doctor's instructions?

☐ Do you feel comfortable asking your doctor for clarification?

If you answered "no" to any of these questions, you may have a problem with your relationship which may stem from your attitude. But, it's my doctor's attitude...the office... the system...you may be saying. In placing the blame on any of these factors outside yourself, even if there is some merit in it, is a prime symptom of an attitude problem – your attitude toward your health care. And worse, it allows you to take on the victim mantle.

"No" answers to any of the above questions should now have you considering the sources of the problem and the first place to look is inside yourself. In doing so, consider the following questions:

☐ Do you read, watch, listen to media reports about healthcare crises?

☐ Do you listen to others when they tell you their own horror stories about their healthcare experiences?

☐ Do you read web sites about health care without checking for credibility?

☐ Have you had a bad experience with the healthcare system in the past?

Just considering these questions should lead you to the conclusion that your own past experiences are in the past, and that whatever anyone else says about health care, they are not the ones there in the midst of your current situation. It is that current situation and the attitude you bring to that encounter that count in the evolution of your relationship with your healthcare providers.

Your own attitude toward health care in general and your own health care in particular will have a powerful effect on the decision you make about your health. Remember that when you are in the role of patient, you are not in control of the entire situation. Your attitude is one thing that you can control.

THE PLACEBO EFFECT

Before we move to the how-to of this chapter – evaluating your own attitude – we need to mention one very powerful effect of your attitude – that is the placebo effect.

For many years, medical researchers have recognized what has come to be known as the placebo effect. The word placebo comes from the Latin word placebo which means "I shall please." A placebo, therefore, has come to mean something – a substance or service perhaps – that is given to a patient to "please" him or her. The dictionary even considers it something to "humour" a patient. Often in medical research, the test group will be provided with the actual treatment under consideration while the control group will be given a placebo: a harmless treatment that should have no medical effect. Then the results from the two groups are compared.

The interesting thing about placebos is that medical researchers know that if a patient believes that the treatment provided will work, a high proportion of them will actually experience that effect despite the placebo having no real medical value. In fact, some 30% of such patients will have the effect they believe it will have. If you were to provide 100 arthritis sufferers with a sugar pill that they were all convinced was a new pain killer specifically for their kind of pain, we could predict quite accurately that about 30 of those patients would likely experience a reduction in pain. Why this happens isn't clear even today with all the interest in the mind-body connection (which we'll discuss in detail in Chapter Four). What we do know is that the patient's attitude toward the treatment is a powerful tool.

> *Give someone who has faith in you a placebo and call it a hair growing pill, anti-nausea pill or whatever, and you will be amazed at how many respond to your therapy.* ~ Bernie Siegel

The bottom line is that if you expect that you will have a good encounter with the healthcare system, if you expect that you will feel better if you follow your doctor's advice, if you expect to have a positive outcome from that herbal remedy you picked up... then you are more likely to do so. A 30% chance of winning is a good reason to have a positive attitude. (Although this is equally a good reason to promote useless products that may actually work for some people – from which the testimonials derive – for these people its effectiveness is 100%.)

MEASURING YOUR ATTITUDE

We've already taken a superficial look at your attitude, but we need to look a bit deeper so that when it comes to figuring out how to fix it, you know what's wrong. Take this test:

Do I Have a Positive Attitude?

I watch the news every day.	_____ yes	_____ no
I read the paper every day.	_____ yes	_____ no
My small talk is often about problems.	_____ yes	_____ no
When I get mad, I stay mad indefinitely.	_____ yes	_____ no
I worry a lot.	_____ yes	_____ no
I often consider the worst that could happen.	_____ yes	_____ no
When the weather is bad, it affects my mood.	_____ yes	_____ no
When things go wrong, it's someone else's fault.	_____ yes	_____ no
I often ask, "Why me?"	_____ yes	_____ no
I usually feel I have no choice in matters.	_____ yes	_____ no

Key to your attitude assessment: Fewer than two yes's means you probably have a generally positive outlook. Three to five yes's means that you had better take a look at that generally negative attitude. If you answered yes to more than half of these questions, you will need to do serious work on your attitude before you can apply common sense to your health.

"FIXING" YOUR ATTITUDE PROBLEMS

No one is positive about everything, but some of us have a generally more negative approach to life than others. All of us could use an attitude boost once in a while. Here are some things you can do to check that attitude and boost it.

- Catch yourself doing something right for a change. Instead of berating yourself for a stupid decision, pat yourself on the back when something goes right. You might even consider a little concrete reward from time to time. At least take note of it. Write it in a journal if you're so inclined.

- Be conscious of and deliberate about your thoughts. You can't think two thoughts at the same time. If you think about more positive things, you won't have room for the negative ones.

- Reconsider how much of the daily news you take in. Most of it is negative and can affect even the most stalwart of us.

- Spend some time in nature. Even a city has nature if you just look for it. You don't have to go far.

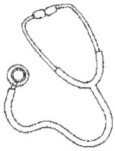

KEYS TO THE LIMITS OF POSITIVE THINKING

☑ Common sense tells us that no one is positive about everything all the time. It isn't human.

☑ Affirmations are only useful to you if they reflect what you believe intellectually and are honest.

☑ Wishing for something isn't the same as believing that you can achieve it.

☑ Understand that your attitudes are painted all over your actions – you can't keep them to yourself.

☑ You need to experience the negative to recognize and cherish the positive.

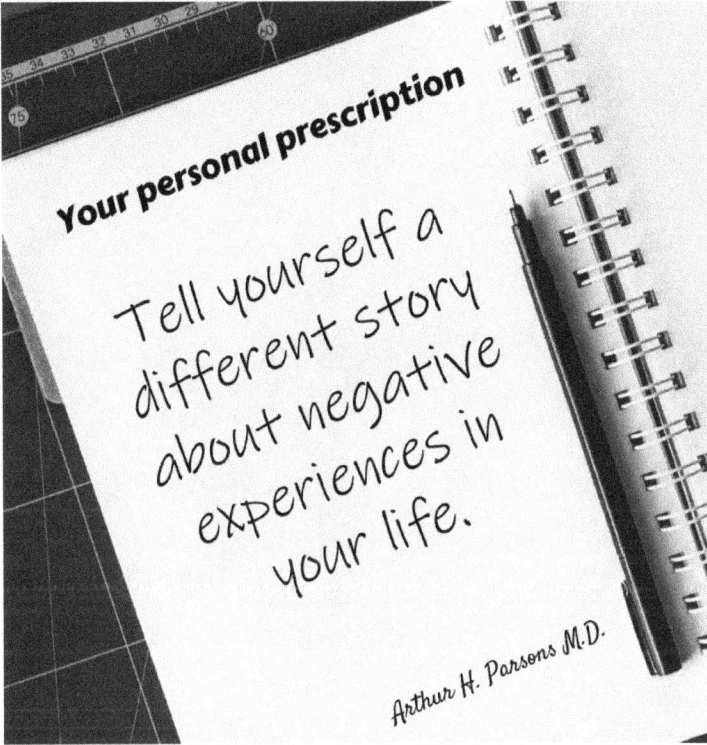

Your personal prescription

Tell yourself a different story about negative experiences in your life.

Arthur H. Parsons M.D.

Parsons

CHAPTER FOUR

SCIENCE AND COMMON SENSE

"Science is a first-rate piece of furniture for a man's upper chamber, if he has common sense on the ground floor."
~ Oliver Wendell Holmes

THERE IS A WIDELY HELD BELIEF in patient circles that mainstream medicine, focused as it appears to be on scientific evidence, is dead set against anything that smacks of "alternative" or "complementary" approaches to health and healing. This might include things like faith healing, holistic medicine, natural medicine, folk medicine, anything unconventional – conventional referring to mainstream medicine. Perhaps even the notion of applying common sense approaches to health issues might fall into one of these categories. After all, in Chapter One I defined common sense as intellect + intuition. Intuition? Isn't that strictly non-scientific? Not really, and I'll tell you why and how in this chapter. But doctors and other mainstream healthcare practitioners aren't the only ones who suffer from this kind of blind faith in science.

Some people, outside the medical community, just simply refuse to believe anything about health and medicine unless they are presented with a scientific explanation. And that scientific approach often comes in the form of more tests, more drugs, more interventions in general, all of which, they believe, are rooted in science. But where that scientific explanation comes from, and how it is interpreted may result in complete misunderstanding. So, let's talk about where science fits into our move toward a common sense approach to your health – and your life

.

WHAT MAKES SOMETHING "SCIENCE"?

Everyone talks about *scientific studies, scientific discoveries, scientific breakthroughs* and so on as if they knew what truly constitutes science – and more that that, what constitutes good science. All you have to do is read, listen or view the news on any given day and you are likely to be confronted with a science-related story. And this story will be related to you by a reporter whose background in science often consists of a fleeting romance with biology classes in the twelfth grade. Can you really trust a news writer, editor or reporter to explain a science story accurately, providing you with the correct interpretation of not only the way the study was designed, but also how it was analysed, how the statistics were arrived at and the conclusions drawn? Before we answer that question, let's take a step back and be sure we all understand what science really means.

There's a years-old comedy piece on YouTube by Irish comic Dara Ó Briain called *Homeopathy and Nutritionists versus Real Medicine*. Ó Briain, who studied mathematics, chemistry and theoretical physics before branching out into comedy, has a few things to say about science. One of his wry observations is his response to people who say to him, "Well, science doesn't know everything." His response: "No, you're right. If science knew everything, IT WOULD STOP!"

[You can see it at https://youtu.be/PnbFgRv8-Kw. It's worth a few minutes of your time]. Science is the beginning, not the end.

Back in Chapter Two we discussed how we develop our beliefs. In that discussion we determined that there are three approaches to acquiring our knowledge and beliefs: *intuition, tenacity, and authority.* We might simply feel that something is correct, or we simply have always believed it to be true, or someone who is an authority to us has told us. You have probably figured out by now that there is also a fourth way: it is called science. And science is a way of thinking, of organizing things and figuring them out – independent of the self. We'll come back to that.

All dictionary definitions of science contain elements of the following:

> ✓ **Science is both a body of knowledge (biological science, medical science and so on) and a process.**
> ✓ **The process of science is systematic: there are specific parameters or rules within which this process takes place.**
> ✓ **Science involves observation and experimentation.**
> ✓ **Science bases its conclusions on observable evidence (rather than opinion or supposition).**

The word "science" itself comes from the Latin *scientia* which means – you guessed it – knowledge. So, when you hear that medicine (or your doctor) is proposing evidence-based solutions to health and disease-related problems, it means that there have been scientific studies conducted using observation and experimentation from which conclusions have been drawn. It means that the conclusions are not someone's opinion or belief – hence, *independent of the self.* Thus, if you are one of those people who needs a scientific explanation before acting on something (such as pursuing a new approach to improving your health), you are not alone: many people feel more comfortable knowing that the approach being suggested is not based on someone's opinion or a celebrity's newest craze (which probably also makes money for her – or him). And the truth is that your personal healthcare provider might also feel more comfortable suggesting something that has more than personal opinion or belief behind it. This is one of the factors behind physicians' and other mainstream healthcare practitioners' skepticism of alternative approaches to health care, many of which lack evidence to support them. So, how can common sense – intellect + intuition – possibly fit into *my* mainstream approach to health and life? Before I get to that, let's go back in time to figure out how science became so important and what impact it has had on how we approach our health and our lives.

Science is a way of thinking much more than it is a body of knowledge. ~ Carl Sagan

SCIENCE: AN EVOLUTION IN HOW TO KNOW THINGS

It is probably safe to say that no one really invented *science*, despite all the Google searches asking that very question. Human beings have been observing their environment and testing out ways of doing things since they first walked the earth. Humans didn't need "science" to discover fire or what it could do, but they did use rudimentary scientific skills to get to the point of being able to roast that wildebeest. So, what we're really talking about is who invented modern science – that is, who invented the scientific method of inquiry as we know it today? Who gave the world that process that is the key to drawing evidence-based conclusions?

Most science historians bestow the honour for having invented science on one man: Francis Bacon. There are some academics and writers who argue that Aristotle, who predated Bacon by centuries, was the inventor of scientific thinking, but it is probably safe to say that, although he did provide us with well-thought-out philosophies that still resonate with us today, if we define science as a process, Sir Francis Bacon gets the prize. Aristotle is probably best categorized as a natural philosopher, a member of an important group of people whose intellectual abilities allowed them to make important observations about the natural world – but they did not use a systematic process. Their contributions are significant, but we need to be clear that science as a way of thinking – a consistent approach to observing and experimenting on phenomena – began much later.

Francis Bacon, who was born in London in 1561, grew up to be a lawyer, a politician and a philosopher, but he was passionate about what we now refer to as empiricism. Empiricism is a philosophy that suggests that knowledge, real knowledge, what we really know, is created through direct observation through our five senses. In other words, if it cannot be observed, it does not exist. This is the basis for the notion that observable phenomena lead to the development of what we now know as the *scientific method*.

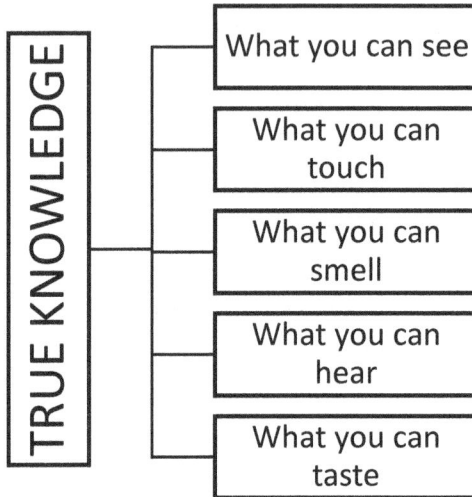

```
                           ┌─────────────────────┐
                    ┌──────│  What you can see   │
                    │      └─────────────────────┘
 ┌─────────┐        │      ┌─────────────────────┐
 │         │        ├──────│  What you can       │
 │  TRUE   │        │      │  touch              │
 │  KNOW-  │        │      └─────────────────────┘
 │  LEDGE  │────────┤      ┌─────────────────────┐
 │         │        ├──────│  What you can       │
 │         │        │      │  smell              │
 │         │        │      └─────────────────────┘
 │         │        │      ┌─────────────────────┐
 │         │        ├──────│  What you can       │
 │         │        │      │  hear               │
 │         │        │      └─────────────────────┘
 │         │        │      ┌─────────────────────┐
 │         │        └──────│  What you can       │
 │         │               │  taste              │
 └─────────┘               └─────────────────────┘
```

So, if true knowledge comes to us only through our five senses, what about God? Well, that's a discussion for another book. In the meantime, let's just follow the history to see if we can put some of those disparate ideas back together. But before we get to that, we need to go a bit further in this exploration of how scientific thinking developed.

THE SCIENTIFIC STUDY: THE GOLD STANDARD OF HOW WE KNOW?

If science is a way of knowing, and it is based on a process, what precisely does that process consist of?

First, it is important to understand that one of the reasons that scientists are so quick to respond to the work of other scientists is that there is an accepted way of applying the scientific process – that is, there is a conventional way of structuring a study and conventional methods for data collection – that is understood world-wide by other scientists. They understand how one another thinks. So, if, from time to time, one of their own decides to take a different path to knowledge, he or she will often be hotly criticized.

The so-called scientific method is really a simple decision-making process. The scientist sees a problem and begins by distilling it down into a clear statement with supporting elements. Often, a problem statement will address the same issues as a good news story is designed to do: *what* is the problem, *why* it's a problem, *who* is affected by it, *where* is the problem located (this broadly includes many areas such as in the healthcare system, in a hospital, in a community, in a part of the body when it comes to research about a disease), *when* the problem occurs or is noticed, and a glimpse of *how* it might be solved.

> *There are in fact two things, science and opinion; the former begets knowledge, the latter ignorance.* ~ Hippocrates

After the problem is succinctly stated, the researcher is well on the way to conducting the research. The second step is the development of a hypothesis. A hypothesis is another statement, but this time it is stated in a very succinct way that articulates precisely what is going to be tested in the subsequent study. The term hypothesis means a supposition, a theory, an untested idea about how the problem might be solved. For example, when researchers are testing a new drug, the hypothesis relates to how they expect the drug will work, based on a limited amount of information to date. It will then be the job of the study itself to collect the data that the researchers will need to determine whether or not their hypothesis – their supposition – is correct or not.

Once they have that hypothesis, the researchers must figure out a way to test that hypothesis – to figure out whether or not their supposition is correct. Although there is plenty of opportunity for errors to be made in any step of the scientific method's process, this is probably the most important key to understanding the quality of a research project. There are several different ways to design a study under the rubric of science, but there is only one that is considered the "gold standard." Before we get to what that means, it's important to understand that just because something is referred to as "scientific research" does not mean it has been designed with that "gold standard" approach – sometimes that isn't even possible.

STEPS IN THE SCIENTIFIC PROCESS

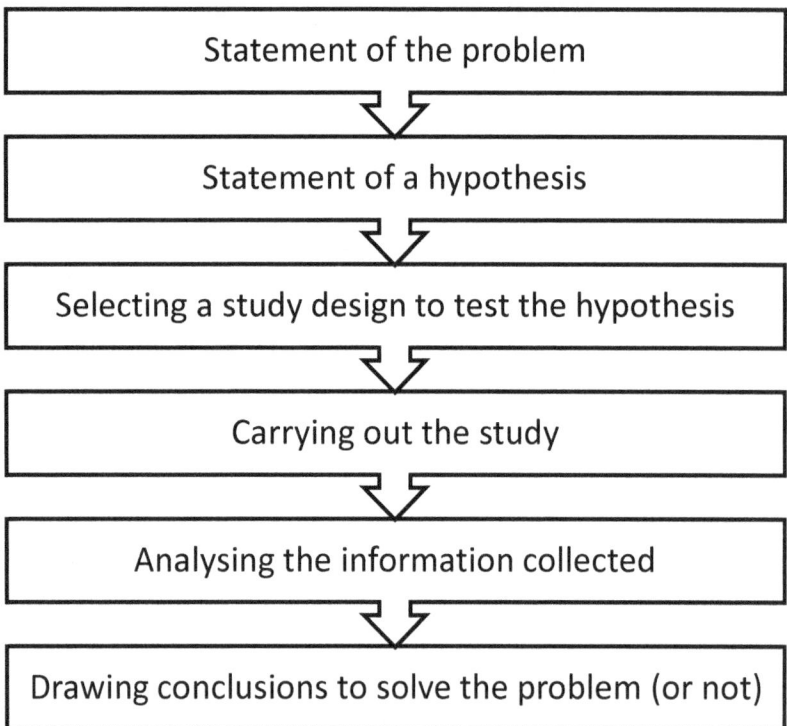

Statement of the problem

Statement of a hypothesis

Selecting a study design to test the hypothesis

Carrying out the study

Analysing the information collected

Drawing conclusions to solve the problem (or not)

There are several acceptable ways that research studies can be designed. Although they are not all equivalent in terms of the strength of their results, different kinds of studies require different kinds of designs after which scientists apply certain kinds of statistical procedures to the data (the results) to figure out how valid these results really are. The kinds of statistical analyses depend on a number of factors including the kind of data – such as data that can be counted versus data that cannot be counted (such as the number of kilometres individual study subjects walk every day, which would have a different mathematical – statistical – test applied to it if the data cannot be counted, such as when people in a research study tell the researchers that they felt good, better or best. This cannot be counted.)

Some of the accepted research designs are as follows:

> ✓ **One-shot case studies**
> ✓ **Case-control studies**
> ✓ **Pre-test-post-test control group studies**
> ✓ **Double-blind randomised control studies (the Gold Standard)**

One-Shot Case Studies: You have probably already heard of the case study. This is where the researcher looks at an individual – this could be a person, or perhaps a group of people or even a particular situation – who meets certain criteria. The case is followed and described to see what happens. Although interesting information can be revealed from these cases, you need to be aware that the conclusions have limitations.

Case studies can stimulate interesting new ideas that researchers then follow up on using other types of more rigorous studies, but the results drawn from individual cases are disputable. One of the biggest problems with case studies is that they cannot be *replicated*, an important concept in scientific research. This means that conducting another study of the same situation and getting similar results is not possible here. A case study is really the systematic formalization of what you often hear about as *anecdotal evidence* – evidence that results from informal observation: anecdotes, stories if you like. We have all observed situations that may be thought provoking, but just because something happened in one situation does not mean that it is able to predict what will happen in all situations. For example, in my medical practice I might have a patient who tells me that he started eating an orange every day and it has improved his sex life. He suggests that I should tell others about his findings. This is an anecdote. If a researcher took this case and made a formal analysis of it, examining all aspects of the patient's life, a case study could be made of it. But I still would not recommend that the way to improve your sex life is to eat an orange every day (although I would recommend that you review the material on placebo effect from Chapter 3. It just might work for you!)

Common sense tells us that we cannot necessarily rely on information that came as a result of an anecdotal observation, and perhaps not even from a formal case study.

Case Control Studies: This is a slightly more vigorous kind of study than a simple case study. In this situation, a case situation is observed and compared to a control case. For example, if you want to study the impact of eating oranges on older adults' sex lives you might gather a group of older adults who never eat oranges then ask them about their sex lives. You would then gather another similar group of older adults each of whom is in the habit of eating an orange every day, then ask them about their sex lives. You then compare the two to see if there are any differences. This seems like a good way to draw conclusions, doesn't it? Well, not really. There are many other factors that could play a part in the sex lives of the individuals in either group: health status, happiness level, marital status, socio-economic status, religious beliefs, cultural norms and so on. You could never be sure it wasn't something else that influenced the results.

Pre-test-post-test Control Group Studies: Now we're getting into the more sophisticated study designs from which more believable results can be gleaned. As the title implies, the design consists of study group and a control group – the study group receives the "treatment" while the control group does not. The expected effects of the "treatment" are measured at the beginning of the study for a benchmark for both groups, then again at the end of the study. The post-test results are compared.

In our study of the effect of oranges on sex lives, we would select similar groups of older adults – ensuring that they are similar in many ways thus reducing the possibility that other factors known as competing *variables*, could be affecting their sex lives. Thus, the groups would be similar in age, socioeconomic status, health status and so on. We would then determine the sex life status of each of the groups. The study group would be administered an orange every day; the control group would not eat oranges for the duration of the test. At the end of the study period, we administer the post-test which is the same as the pre-test and look to see if there are any changes. If our hypothesis that eating an orange every day improves your sex life is correct, we should see an improvement in the sex lives of the members of the study group, but no change in the sex lives of the control group. The question at this point is this: how much of a difference is an important difference? That can only be answered by applying statistical analyses on the study data. We'll get to that later in this chapter.

But pre-test-post-test control group designs are not all the same. There are two fundamental types of studies, and one is the "gold standard", the other is not.

One of the fundamental concepts in this type of study is the extent to which *chance* plays a role in the results. Is it not possible for the results to simply be a matter of chance? Isn't it possible that it is just a coincidence that the people in the study group ended up having better sex than those in the control group? Yes, if the members of the study group are permitted to self-select, it is certainly possible that the improvement in their sex lives is a chance occurrence. That's why researchers talk about *randomized control studies*. In other words, the participants are randomly assigned to one group or the other. This is getting close to the gold standard, but we're not quite there.

The Gold Standard - The double-blind, randomized control study: This is the holy grail of scientific study designs that should inspire the most confidence in their results. This is a sub-type of the randomized, pre-test-post-test control group study, but in this instance, none of the study participants know if they are actually in the study group or in the control group. In our oranges/sex life study, the subjects would not know whether we were testing the effects of apples or oranges. The control group would be fed apples and the study group oranges, but they would not know that we are testing oranges. That's the first part of the blinding. What makes it a *double-blind study* is that in this study design, the researchers themselves would not know which group any of the participants is in either. This is what makes this kind of study so reliable, and so difficult to conduct in many cases. It is this difficulty which often makes researchers default to a less robust type of study design. But as a consumer, it's important that you know the difference. (More on that later.) This design minimizes *bias* – an important concept in the tainting of study results. In our oranges and sex life study, we, as the researchers, would stay at arm's length from the study participants.

We might hire research nurses, for example, to provide the study group participants with their pieces of fruit – and remember, the study participants themselves are unaware of whether they are receiving the test fruit or not. This at least equalizes the possibility of placebo effect in both the study group and the control group which makes the analysis of any differences in the results to be deemed to be based on the treatment – the orange consumption.

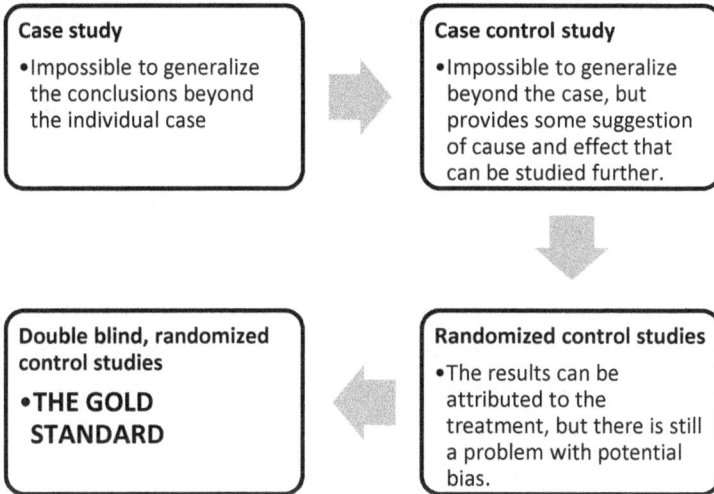

Case study
•Impossible to generalize the conclusions beyond the individual case

Case control study
•Impossible to generalize beyond the case, but provides some suggestion of cause and effect that can be studied further.

Double blind, randomized control studies
•**THE GOLD STANDARD**

Randomized control studies
•The results can be attributed to the treatment, but there is still a problem with potential bias.

Summary: So why is it important that you know anything at all about the way scientific studies are designed? From a common sense perspective, it seems nonsensical for you to read a study or hear about it on the radio or online, then to believe the results (or disbelieve them) if you have no idea of whether or not it is a well-designed study. It is nonsensical for you to believe that you know enough simply by accepting the blogger, reporter, tweeter, celebrity or anyone else's opinion on the importance of a study unless you trust that the person at least knows about science and study design. That is almost always not the case unless the person is a scientist. If you are still sceptical, let's talk a bit about the misrepresentation of science.

MISUSE AND MISINTERPRETATION OF SCIENCE THROUGH STATISTICS

Understanding scientific data might not be the be all and end all of knowledge that we need to help us along on our life's journey, but not knowing when you are being fed misleading, inaccurate information can make things worse. Let's look at some ways that science and scientific research are being misused and misinterpreted.

Earlier in this chapter I talked about the fact that after researchers gather up the results from their study and control groups, they then apply appropriate mathematical procedures to the data before they report their conclusions. Even if you know nothing about statistics, you have probably heard things like the following: sample size, margin of error, correlation, confidence level, variables, bias, cause and effect etc. These are all statistical terms that are frequently used when research studies are being reported on, whether in news feeds, on blogs, on television, or online. And they are all terms that make many people's eyes glaze over. They simply stop listening when someone begins to discuss the margin of error in a research study. But they are very important elements in helping you to determine whether or not you should sit up and pay attention to the results—whether or not there is important information for you here. This boredom with the statistical analyses of research data is one of the more important factors in how science is misrepresented and misused. Since there is far too much information to go into here (and your eyes would soon glaze over), let's focus on four obvious signs that science is being misrepresented to you.

WHY SCIENCE DOESN'T "PROVE" THINGS

How many times have you heard something like this: "This product is clinically *proven* to improve your insomnia..." or "Scientific studies have *proven* that our toothpaste works better than our competitor's..." Does or can a scientific study *prove* anything? The startling truth is that scientific "proof" if not precisely a myth, is an almost impossible conclusion in most studies. So, what does it mean to prove something?

Generally speaking, proving something requires that it demonstrates the truth, the truth being, contrary to what we might be led to believe these days, *in accordance with reality*. To prove something in scientific terms means that there can be absolutely *no doubt whatsoever* that it could be wrong. But, as we have demonstrated in our discussion of the design of research studies, there is generally plenty of room for doubt, however small, because of the inability of scientists to disprove any and all competing explanations for the outcome of a study. There are few studies reported in

Statistical thinking will one day be as necessary for efficient citizenship as the ability to read and write. ~ H.G.Wells

the media and online that are iron-clad and can actually be deemed to prove anything. What they can do, however, is *provide evidence that can demonstrate strongly*. And evidence is important.

Having evidence of something is far better than the alternative: misinformation circulated by individuals of dubious expertise based on little more than *their personal opinions*. When we put it in these terms, it does seem a bit nonsensical to accept health recommendations from celebrities, neighbours, even well-meaning friends, without evidence to support their advice, doesn't it?

Even scientists themselves will tell you that the process of conducting scientific research involves collecting data to support their predictions – what we have already described as the hypothesis part of the scientific method.

So, if you are faced with a study that reports that it "proves" something, common sense would tell you that it may, in fact, demonstrate the effect, but it is unlikely that it proves it. You need to know more about the strength of the conclusion. This is useful information for you in making a decision whether or not to act on those study results.

THE FALLACY OF "REGRESSION TO THE MEAN"

This is less complicated than it sounds. And it is a way that events or phenomena are explained far too often. What it means is that an event or occurrence is deemed to be the direct result of something simply because it occurred right after. For example, if I have a patient who comes into my office and tells me that he ate an orange and his migraine went away leading him to conclude that oranges cure migraine headaches, this is a fallacy. The orange cannot be construed to be the migraine cure, despite one individual's personal experience. Further, should he try to market oranges as a cure for migraines, he is on precarious ground indeed. And if you hear a news story suggesting oranges as a migraine cure based on this data, you are listening to a report that is inaccurate at best, and probably downright deceitful. Remember, though, if a patient believes strongly that oranges cure his personal headaches, he is likely to see that effect some 30% of the time – remember the placebo effect.

EX POST FACTO INFERENCE

This is another fallacy that is similar to the previous one, and just as simple to understand. It refers to drawing conclusions after the fact – that is, there has been no proactive research done, only conclusions about the cause and effect relationship between naturally occurring phenomena. The most famously used example of an *ex post facto* inference is the following.

One year, storks were observed in large numbers in a Swedish town. The number of births at the local maternity hospital increased all during the time that the storks were in residence in the town. Therefore, storks bring babies. Nonsense? Of course, but it is an example of the kind of cause and effect relationships that can be drawn if we are not careful about the research design and how the statistics are applied.

SCIENCE PROGRESSES IN MICRO-STEPS – NOT IN BREAKTHROUGHS

It's often easy to conclude that every time a scientific story is conveyed in the media that it is a major breakthrough that will immediately improve the health and lives of hundreds if not thousands of people. But the truth of the matter is that science progresses slowly. Even so-called breakthroughs are usually the result of painstaking work carried out over years if not decades. So much of the scientific progress you read about in the news, if it looks like a major breakthrough, it's important to do a bit of digging to figure out (a) if it is really a breakthrough, and (b) if it is meaningful.

THE MEDIA'S ROLE IN SCIENTIFIC MISREPRESENTATION

It should be clear to you by now, that the way science is reported in the media – whether traditional media like television news shows, or online – is not always truthful, accurate or even important. Sometimes it is simply a result of the way the statistics are reported by a journalist who does not understand them or cannot

Facts are stubborn, but statistics are more pliable. ~ Mark Twain

convey them well, or it is simply that a science story isn't as important as it sounds. But there are two other issues that you need to consider when applying common sense to what you are exposed to via the media both traditional and online: the media's use of scientists themselves, and oversimplification of science.

Old public relations people often suggest that if they have a something that they want to convince you of, they don't even entertain the idea of telling you directly. (I know this because my wife is an old PR person.) They hire someone you, the consumer, find credible, then they put their words into that person's mouth. This is called third-party endorsement and it has been around ever since there have been people who need to persuade you of something. One of those groups of third-party endorsers consists of scientists, which, when it comes to health-related stories, often includes physicians. You would believe a scientist, wouldn't you?

There are three aspects to the answer to the question.

First, can't you believe it if the scientist is talking about his or her own research? The answer is a resounding maybe. Although it is highly likely that the scientist, and this includes medical scientists, will tell you the "truth", it is only one version of the truth. (Later on in the book I'll talk more about the concept of *framing* a story, but for now let's just simply define it as looking at a story from only one specific aspect thus omitting other aspects that might provide a more comprehensive perspective.) Sometimes, scientists or their publicity people, select only one aspect of the story to tell.

Second, and this is very common, the scientist tells his or her story to a journalist who in turn reports it, often selecting only the most newsworthy – in his or her view – aspects. The scientist has no control over what facts the journalist emphasizes, or how the story is slanted. So often the public thinks that the story was provided by the scientist that way, but creative editing on the part of the news outlet (or online blogger) can create a different story indeed – a situation over which the scientist has no say. Often this kind of selective reporting can be deceptive, even if the words came from the scientist. The story has now acquired not only the scientist's bias, but also the bias of the news writer and editor. Common sense tells us that it might not be completely accurate.

Finally, it's important to understand that some (perhaps many) of the physicians you see being interviewed in the news are what you might call "paid shills." In other words, they have been paid by drug companies or medical device manufacturers to provide their "expert" opinions. This payment is often not as evident as you might hope it to be. For example, the doctor will not likely be on the drug company payroll; rather he or she will have been wined and dined or paid for his or her consulting expertise of one sort or another. The fact that the information presented by that physician might have been influenced by an outside party that has a monetary interest in the acceptance of the story as truth ought to change your perspective on believing it. Or at least compel you to develop a healthy skepticism.

THE DANGERS OF OVER SIMPLIFYING SCIENCE

Science can often seem difficult to understand. It uses vocabulary that we don't use in everyday life; it seems to require a complex knowledge of biology, chemistry and physics to name just three major scientific areas; it seems to follow complicated methods. When intermediaries such as journalists, or even more problematic, celebrities present science, they try to simplify it. The problem is that in the process of trying to make science understandable to others, often important elements are dropped, thus changing the story. Excellent science communicators, however, have such a deep understanding of both science and communication that they are able to select the important aspects of a science story and convey it in a way that people without a science background can understand.

The trouble is, that there are so few truly talented science communicators. What we often have is a collection of reporters and celebrities who become the face of the science story often resulting in misinformation that those reading or listening use to base health decisions on. This doesn't make a lot of sense, and yet it continues.

Over the past decade, we have all been treated to the development of what has become known as "The CSI" effect. You are probably familiar with the television franchise knowns as CSI (Crime Scene Investigation). Their stock in trade from the very beginning has been to portray over-the-top forensic science in such a way that in the real world the public has begun to expect that kind of scientific evidence – even on juries. In reality, however, the technology is not as sophisticated or definitive. This expectation that science in the real world will emulate science in fictional television or movies spills out over into other types of science such as medical science. And this kind of over-simplification of what is really very complex can lead to misinformation.

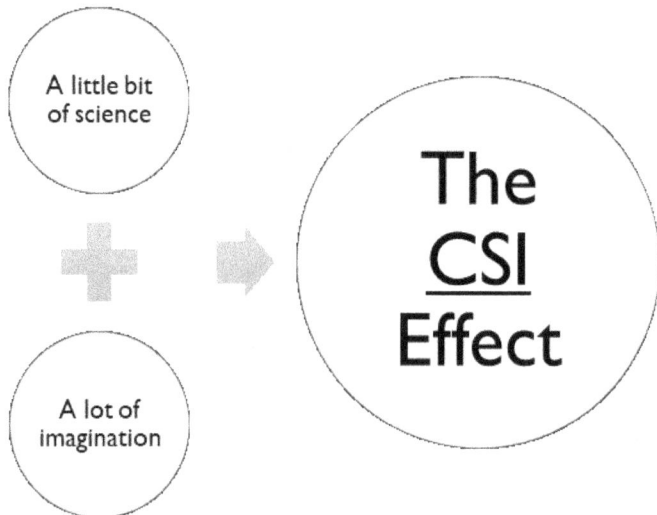

Too much imagination with your little bit of science can lead to an over-simplification of what science can offer you. Now that you understand a bit about scientific inquiry, and the problem with truth and facts, let's turn our attention to the science of common sense.

RENÉ DESCARTES AND HIS MIND-BODY DISCONNECTION

To begin to understand how common sense can have a basis in science, we have to go back in history to visit with René Descartes.

How you categorize Descartes depends on whose work you read, and how you read it. If you read about him from a philosophical perspective, you will get one view. If you read him from a mathematical perspective, the story will be different. Objectively speaking, René Descartes was a seventeenth century mathematician, physician and philosopher (with a law degree in there for good measure) whose work was influential during his lifetime and continues to resonate with us today.

Often referred to as the founder of modern philosophy, Descartes has had a profound impact on how modern medicine views the human condition. In fact, we are only now in recovery from his view. And here's why we need to recover from his philosophical approach to medicine and healing.

One of Descartes's most enduring contributions to how we think about ourselves resulted from his desire to create a method that would find the "truth." Sound familiar? These days, there would seem to be nothing more important than discerning the truth of just about anything. It is quite likely that you are already familiar with the fundamental teaching of his philosophy and don't know it.

Cogit ergo sum. No? How about, "I think, therefore I am." That one is probably very familiar to you. This was a theme of much of his work. In the original French it was, *"Je pense, donc je suis."* This is what Descartes believed was the fundamental way in which we obtain knowledge. But his belief in the relationship – or should we say the separation – between the mind and the body is arguably the most problematic concept in how modern medicine is practiced, and how modern health care is delivered.

According to René Descartes, our minds are completely distinct from our bodies: one has no impact on the other. Consider for a moment what this would really mean in health terms. It means that anything you believe about the physical effects of stress for example, are completely false. Descartes would say, "It's all in your head." And this point of view permeated medical diagnosis and treatment for several hundred years. And if you think about how difficult it is to change entrenched ideas, you may be slightly more sympathetic to the medical community in their difficulty in accepting the mind-body connection that was revisited in the 20th century and that has changed our way of dealing with any number of health and disease conditions.

He also believed that "science must be founded on certainty…" And we have already discussed the extent to which science is not all that certain at all. So, if Descartes has been so influential, who has come along to help us back to understanding that the mind and the body are, indeed, connected, and it is this connection that provides us with our common sense?

TURNING DESCARTES ON HIS HEAD: PUTTING MIND AND BODY BACK TOGETHER

Over the centuries the medical/scientific community has largely resisted change. This has been the case since the days of Copernicus, the sixteenth century astronomer who postulated that the sun rather than the earth was at the centre of the universe, turning the accepted science upside down. Thus, many of the advocates for change have had to leave the scientific fold one way or another: sometimes they left of their own accord; other times they were forced out. But what happens to scientists who leave the path of traditional science? Sometimes they continue their work outside the traditional boundaries of science, *eventually* making contributions that *eventually* are accepted by their former colleagues. Other times, however, they continue their work, promoting it and publishing on the fringes, without the checks and balances provided by the scientific community. The twenty-first century has provided the technology to make it much easier for these charlatans to get their ideas into the public mindset all under the veneer of legitimate scientific credentials. No where has the problem of pseudoscience been more fraught than in this area of mind-body medicine. *Caveat emptor*. Buyer beware.

In any case, there have been mainstream scientists whose work in more recent years has turned conventional thinking upside down. Several of them are important to understanding a common sense approach to health.

TYPE A BEHAVIOUR AND YOUR HEART: FRIEDMAN AND ROSENMAN

After René Descartes did a good job of convincing generations of medical practitioners that there is a complete separation between the mind and the body, groups of medical researchers, not to mention patients, have been trying to put these two notions back together since American cardiologists Meyer Friedman and R.H. Rosenman presented their findings on what they called type A behaviour and its contribution to heart disease in the 1970's.

For centuries, even throughout the years of Descartes-influenced medical care, people have subscribed to the idea that there is, and has always been, a relationship between our emotions and our hearts.

You might say, "He was heart-broken," or perhaps, "The letter was heart-felt," or, "The widow was heart-sore." All these phrases suggest that our hearts somehow are at the seat of our emotions. Although this is not a reference to the science behind grief or sadness, it does speak to a long-held view of the connection between mind (emotions in this case), and body. In fact, one of the earliest references in the medical literature that suggested this relationship was written in 1812 by Napoléon Bonaparte's personal physician Jean-Nicolas Corvisart where he attributed heart disease to "actions of the organ and passions of the mind." So, this is not a new idea.

It was during the middle of the twentieth century that the effects of personality and specific behavioural characteristics on heart health really began to find a place in scientific research. The personality type that was first associated with higher than average risk of heart disease is now well known to us. Some of the attributes, as you likely already know, are a strong drive to succeed, a lack of satisfaction with this success, aggressiveness and a preoccupation with time.

Until 1959 when Friedman and Rosenman began their long-term prospective study, the evidence to support this relationship was based on retrospective studies of patients who had already suffered a myocardial infarction – a heart attack. Of course, after our discussion of well-designed research studies, you can probably see that in this kind of study, you would be hard pressed to figure out which came first: the personality traits or the heart disease since you're only looking at patients who have already suffered that heart attack. Friedman and Rosenman took a prospective approach, beginning their research by following 209 male business executives and physicians. They controlled for diet, tobacco and alcohol consumption and found that the average serum cholesterol was much higher in those with what Friedman and Rosenman now described as "Type A" personalities, a phrase that is very familiar to anyone who is interested in heart disease. In addition, coronary heart disease was seven times more frequent in the group exhibiting these personality characteristics.

The follow-up study of the group continued for years, the results only further confirming the original hypothesis that heart disease was at least in part tied to stress and personality characteristics. Since that time, many more sophisticated studies have provided further supporting evidence. By 1973 researchers were focusing on the relationship specifically between stress and heart disease, rather than a simple list of pre-determined personality characteristics.

Since that ground-breaking research, the medical community has begun to see that there is truly a relationship between the mind and the body, but that didn't mean that the centuries of Descartes' influence had been erased. There was still a long way to go and much of that work was done by scientists who had to buck the mainstream.

CANDACE PERT & MOLECULES OF EMOTION

It would take a well-regarded neuroscientist to turn the tables on mainstream medicine. Dr. Candace Pert, who died in 2013, was one of the discoverers of opioid receptors in the brain, a truly significant contribution to how we understand how drugs work. Interestingly, this work led to a Nobel prize but not for her: she was only one of several bench scientists working in the lab and was not cited in the publication of the research findings. In any event, it was, however, not this work that she was known for by the time she died.

In the foreword to her most popular book *Molecules of Emotion: The Science Behind Mind-Body Medicine*, Deepak Chopra wrote the following:

"Her pioneering research has demonstrated how our internal chemicals, the neuropeptides and their receptors, are the actual biological underpinnings of our awareness, manifesting themselves as our emotions, beliefs and expectations, and profoundly influencing how we respond to and experience the world."

Her scientific work connected, even for the most sceptical medical-scientific among us, actual, demonstrable physiological reactions to our emotional responses, our beliefs, our attitudes – our minds. The science behind this connection begins with the molecular receptor that she helped to discover early in her career: the opiate receptor. There have been many such receptors for other substances discovered since that time. When a receptor receives a message initiated by a specific molecule docking with it, that information then goes deep within the body of the cell where the message, whatever it is, can radically alter the cell resulting in physical cell changes.

I'm a scientist. We don't talk about the spirit. Soul is a four-letter word in our tradition. ~ Dr. Candace Pert

She then moved on to examining peptides which are short chains of amino acids that are the basic building blocks of proteins. These proteins are widely distributed in the body in the form of substances such as hormones and neurotransmitters, to name only two, but she prefers to refer to them as "informational substances" or messenger molecules that distribute information throughout the body. In this way, they become what she further refers to as the biochemicals of emotion since they can be produced by psycho-emotional events, they can be stored in various parts of the body and they can then have dramatic impacts on physical well-being.

Her work was based on her hypothesis that all illness has at least some psychosomatic component. In her 1997 book *Molecules of Emotion*, which I mentioned earlier, she tells the story of how her work was considered to be far outside the mainstream of medical research, reiterating the fact that truly ground-breaking ideas have rarely been welcomed in science (remember our reference to Copernicus earlier in this chapter?). Her research was advocating a more *holistic* approach to health and disease care, an approach that was somewhat radical when she first began working on it. Holistic, as an approach to health, is a notion that is so ubiquitous in our society these days, that we seem to have forgotten what it really means – and what it meant to Dr. Pert. It means treating the whole of someone, not just a part. Not just treating a person's heart or liver or stomach but seeing that as a part of a whole. Holistic does not mean alternative, or offbeat or complementary or unorthodox. It simply means whole. However, mainstream medicine saw it in less flattering terms.

BRUCE LIPTON AND THE BIOLOGY OF BELIEF

It should be clear to you by now that I believe that there is a direct connection between attitudes/beliefs/emotions and physical health, and that there is good science to support this link. Before we move on, there is one more researcher/practitioner whose work I believe provides even further support for common sense and health. That contributor is American stem cell biologist, Dr. Bruce Lipton.

Another scientist whose views were often the opposite of widely supported approaches in mainstream medicine, Dr. Lipton's main hypothesis was that the behaviour of our cells is controlled by factors in the cell's environment, including polypeptides produced by our emotions. When information from these factors make its way through the cell membrane, certain genes can be turned on and off. Mainstream science had already concluded that genes are static and are the controllers of cell destiny as it were. Although mainstream science continues to consider Dr. Lipton's work to be fringe, at best, he provides evidence of tantalizing scientific connections between emotions and the way our genes express themselves – evidence that is too important to ignore.

Dr. Lipton's work suggests that our genes may not, in fact, be our destiny, but that, as he says in his 2005 book *The Biology of Belief*, "Environmental influences, including nutrition, stress and emotions, can modify those genes without changing their basic blueprint..." and further, that these can then be transmitted to future generations. The mechanism by which this happens is a complex physiological one rooted in protein synthesis which he describes in his book. Fundamentally, he believes that our cells are not controlled by their nuclei as has long been believed, rather by their environments, and further, that it is the cell membrane that plays the most important role. His suggestion that cell behaviour is based on a variety of elements – what he describes as a holistic way of viewing them – is a bit of a microcosm analogy to Dr. Pert's holistic approach to the entire body.

In my view, if the mind and body are viewed as separate, it gives us an excuse for not taking responsibility for our own health and well-being. It lets us off the hook. It is the easy way out, an approach to life that it seems many, if not most, modern humans prefer.

THE BOTTOM LINE FOR SCIENCE & COMMON SENSE

Carl Sagan once said: "We live in a society exquisitely dependent on science and technology, in which hardly anyone knows anything about science and technology." That is more than ever true about our health and the health care we seek to support it.

It has been demonstrated that a one-cell organism that does not have a central nervous system (or brain) will avoid noxious substances and approach substances that nourish them.

If a single-cell has this common sense to avoid what is harmful, then it stands to reason that we, as human beings, have a higher form of common sense – after all, we are a collection of billions of cells. The early one-celled organisms could be in either growth or protection mode; they could not do both simultaneously. For human beings, common sense is important for both personal protection and as a force for growth.

A common sense approach to your health is based on first understanding that you don't really comprehend the basis of everything, the appreciation of which should compel you to seek ways to improve that knowledge. If there is a relationship between your mind and your body, then how you think about your health and what you understand about it will have a dramatic impact on the outcomes. Again, remember the placebo effect?

Even as much of mainstream medicine continues to criticize some of the work done by mind-body medicine specialists, there is no denying their own contention that 30% of the time that you believe a treatment will work, it probably will. That's the most fundamental and widely accepted mind-body connection. What you need to know as you take a common sense approach to your own health, is that there is probably a more significant connection than you may have considered. As we work through some of the situations where a common sense approach is warranted, the connection between what you think and how you feel is key.

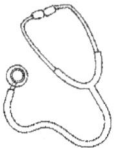

KEYS TO USING SCIENCE AS A BASIS FOR COMMON SENSE

☑ Understand that if something is too good to be true, it probably is.

☑ Be aware that science is often misused by the media.

☑ Pay attention to how scientific studies are presented to you and by whom.

☑ Check the credibility of sources of medical scientific information.

☑ Remember that science doesn't prove things; it provides evidence.

☑ Understand that your mind and body are intimately connected.

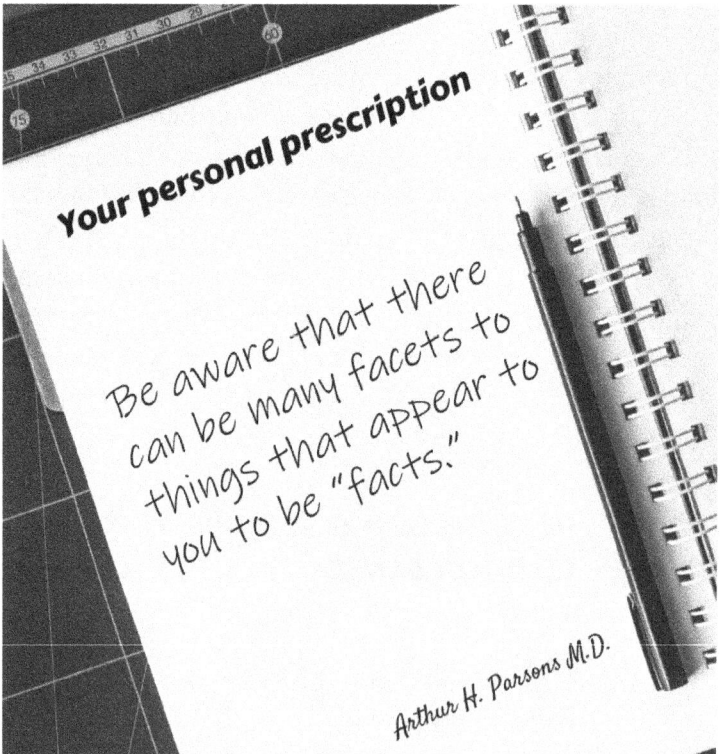

Your personal prescription

Be aware that there can be many facets to things that appear to you to be "facts."

Arthur H. Parsons M.D.

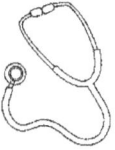

MEANWHILE, BACK IN THE OFFICE

PETE HAD NOW BEEN ON THE JOB FOR SIX MONTHS. It was Friday afternoon and he was feeling more than a bit tired. His two nights on call this past week had been very busy, so he hadn't had as much sleep as he might have wanted in order to be on top of his game. As he poured himself a cup of coffee to take to his desk, better to face the afternoon's slate of patients, he was thinking about the steep learning curve he was on. Who knew that four years in medical school followed by a two-year family medicine residency would still leave him with the feeling that he didn't know quite as much as he ought to? On the whole, perhaps it was better that he realized this, rather than thinking he knew everything. He took a deep breath and patted his pocket where his smartphone nestled. *What did doctors ever do before apps?* he wondered. More than a few times over the past several months, referring to his favourite drug reference app had ensured that he wrote out the correct dosage on those prescription pads.

"She's in your examining room," Tara whispered as Pete walked past the reception desk on his way to see his next patient.

The "she" to whom Tara referred was a 46-year-old woman named Amelia Donaldson. A bank teller, Amelia was married with two children and a penchant for every new-fangled medical test she read about or heard about – and make no mistake, she read and listened to everyone. On her last visit she had informed him in no uncertain terms that she needed some kind of test that Dr. Oz had recommended on his television show. According to him, backed up by such other medical expertise as actor/entrepreneur and self-styled wellness guru Gwyneth Paltrow, every woman over the age of 40 required it annually. Pete couldn't even remember now what it was since it was the third or fourth time she had appeared in his office in a matter of eight weeks looking for various tests, none of which she actually needed.

Pete dropped his now-empty coffee mug in his office, took a deep breath and went next door to his examining room.

Amelia was sitting primly on the examining table – most patients took a seat in a chair – the better to be ready to whip out whatever part of her anatomy she was complaining about this week. Pete occasionally worried that one day she might actually have something wrong with her and he'd miss it in the morass of complaints and demands that regularly accompanied her visits.

"Hello Mrs. Donaldson. How are you today?" The minute the question was out of his mouth he was already regretting it. Hadn't he learned yet that this kind of open-ended question just begged for patients like Amelia to begin an unfocused tirade? He should have asked her what specific issue brought her to the office this afternoon. But she was already off and running.

This time it was not a test she was demanding. She had seen an advertisement for a new drug that was purported to be the magic bullet to treat hypothyroidism, the one medical condition that she actually did have. Of course, the source of the information on the magic nature of this new drug was the drug company that produced and sold the drug.

She waved a piece of paper at him. "I printed this out for you," she was saying. "According to the internet, it is much better than that old Synthroid® I've been on for the past three years. I think I should have the latest drug."

Pete sat down at the computer terminal where he quickly brought up her chart. What he really wanted to do was tell her to go stuff it, that she was on the long-standing gold-standard of thyroid medications, and that newer didn't necessarily mean better, but he'd get to that – eventually. "Well, let's see," he said scrolling through her last few blood reports. "I see that your thyroid levels are normal." He turned toward her. "How are you feeling? Any change in your health?"

"I feel perfectly fine," she said snarkily, "no thanks to you."

Life is Terminal

Pete had no idea what she meant by that remark, but he carried on in as professional a manner as he could muster. He proceeded to carry out a physical examination – blood pressure, pulse, palpation of her thyroid.

"So, you're feeling perfectly fine. Your thyroid levels are well-controlled. Your current medication is working well and not causing you any side effects. I have no medical reason to consider changing your medication."

"Well," she said sitting up straighter, "I want the new one."

"It's a lot more expensive than the one you're on," Pete said realizing that the medical reasoning wasn't working.

"I don't care. My health insurance will pay for it."

"You do know that if everyone used the more expensive drugs when the basic ones are working that the insurance rates go up for everyone?"

"Do I look like I care?"

She did not.

"Well, doctor, are you going to give me the prescription I need or not?"

"Of course. You can certainly continue on the drug that you need," he was careful to emphasize the need, "but to tell you the truth, I'm not comfortable changing your medication simply because you *want* it changed when your medical condition is stable and well-controlled. There is no medical indication for a change of any kind at this point."

It was crystal clear to Pete that she was furious, and he was left wondering why anyone bothered to go to medical school when so many of the patients seemed to think they knew better.

"So, you're not giving me this new drug?"

"I'm sorry, Mrs. Donaldson, you simply don't need it and it would not be good medicine on my part if I changed your drug regimen."

95

"Don't need it?" she was beginning to shriek. "Who are you to tell me what I *need*?"

Pete was getting angry. If he wasn't the one to tell her what she needed medically, who was?

"You do not have a medical need for this new drug," Pete said getting up and heading toward the door.

"Where are you going?" she demanded. "I'm not finished."

~

The following Monday morning he was catching his breath between patients when Dr. Kramer's white coat whipped by his open office door. A split second later, Dr. Kramer had turned around and was standing in Pete's doorway.

"Pete," he said, "we haven't had much time to catch up over the past few weeks. How did you fare with that young patient with that unusual rash on his chin we were conferring about?"

"Oh my god," he said. "They don't tell us about those kinds of things in med school. It turns out the kid had a fetish for sucking on drinking glasses."

Dr. Kramer furrowed his brow. "You mean he did it to himself?"

Pete nodded, and they both laughed. "Yeah. It seems he likes to get them suction-cupped to his face." to his face." Then Pete got serious. "Dr. Kramer, do you by any chance have a few minutes to talk?"

Dr. Kramer looked at his watch. "It seems I might have about fifteen minutes." He came into the office closing the door behind him. "What's on your mind?" he said taking the seat across the desk from Pete. "And by the way... I think it's time you started calling me Tony."

Pete had spent the weekend thinking about Amelia Donaldson. On one hand, she had made him furious with her strident demands for the newest and the shiniest. But what really bothered him was the fact that she didn't seem to trust his medical judgment. He felt personally slighted, and it occurred to him that this might not be the healthiest way to approach patients. He just couldn't seem to get over it.

He explained all of this to Dr. Kramer – Tony – who listened closely then sat back in his chair.

"You know, Pete, you remind me a lot of myself when I first started practice."

This seemed like a good thing to Pete. It meant that he was not likely the only one who felt this way. And he couldn't really talk to his med school friends about it since most of them were still effectively in school, opting for longer residencies in other specialties.

Although not really "old" – Tony was in his early 50's – Pete's new partner had over 25 years as a family physician under his belt. He certainly must have learned a thing or two. "Well, I remember going home most nights that first couple of years feeling as if I didn't know what I didn't know, and that sometimes scared me. But as time went on, and I gained self-confidence, I realized that I did know a lot. More than I gave myself credit for quite often. Anyway, the most important thing I learned was that in any medical specialty you have to recognize when you truly don't have the expertise in something."

"Lack of expertise doesn't seem to bother most patients these days," Pete grumbled almost under his breath.

"Excuse me?"

"I mean, so many of the patients who come in these days seem to think that all those celebrities and blogs written by anyone and everyone with an opinion on a health issue, are the experts. Why do they even come to see us?"

Tony laughed. "Well, you've hit the nail on the head it seems. Things have changed a lot in the last 25 years – some things are better; some things are worse. Those patients who come in demanding every new and often ill-advised treatment and test are actually using you for access into the healthcare system. I know it can feel abusive, but you just have to base your decisions on best medical practice and evidence. Sometimes we have to say no to them. But if they're really fixated on something, they'll try to find another doctor who will humour them. I'm not saying it's right. I'm just saying that's what happens."

Pete thought about this for a minute. "When I think about it, most of my patients aren't like that, but the ones who are just seem to overshadow the great relationships I'm developing with so many of them."

"Hold tight to that thought, Pete. Those relationships will be the most important part of your patient's healthcare over the course of their lives. And that's what will give you the most satisfaction." He looked at his watch. "Any other *bon mots* I can provide for you today, Pete?"

"Just the answer to one question, if you could, Tony. Do you have any advice to help me help so many of my patients who seem to like to see themselves as victims?"

Tony stood up, slung his stethoscope over his shoulder and smiled. "That's a tough one, Pete. I think it might require dinner and a beer. Next week?"

CHAPTER FIVE

BE CAREFUL WHAT YOU SAY...EVEN TO YOURSELF

"A word is dead when it is said. Some say. I say it just begins to live that day." ~ Emily Dickinson

IN THE BEGINNING WAS THE WORD, and the word was with God, and the word was God... (John 1:1.). Even if you are not the slightest bit religious, or have any interest in the Christian bible, you have probably heard this line before. But have you ever really thought about what it means – in secular terms? Words are powerful things. They are arguably the building blocks of our personal universe. Our words, what labels we put on things, and the way we use them, establish a basic foundation for the actions we will eventually take in our search for high quality health care.

Words are fundamental to our ability to communicate. And how we communicate to others says a lot about us as individuals in the world. However, and perhaps even more important, is how we communicate with ourselves. The words we use to describe ourselves and our world, even if we never say one word out loud, create a frame around us, providing both boundaries and opportunities.

So, both the words we use in communication with others, as well as the words we use in our own internal dialogue, have a profound effect on our health and well-being. A common sense approach to getting to optimal health suggests that it's important to choose our words carefully.

HOW ARE YOU? BE CAREFUL HOW YOU ANSWER

It's such a common phrase, we often fail to even hear it before we mindlessly respond.

"I'm okay." "Fine." "Still alive." "I've been better." "I've been worse."

What about, "Great!"

When you look at each of these automatic responses, doesn't it seem that each of them says something different about the individual uttering them? In each case the response tells a story to the person asking after your health; each of these responses also tells *you* a story. And make no mistake, hearing yourself saying these words out loud is even more powerful than your internal dialogue. If you have never thought about it before, it's time to think carefully about how you as an individual habitually respond when someone asks the simple question, "How are you?"

Words are, of course, the most powerful drug used by mankind. ~ Rudyard Kipling

It's small talk, you say. It's a conversation starter that is not designed to be about anything important. Yes, of course, by definition that is quite accurate. But it's dangerous to underestimate the impact of small talk such as that referring to your personal well-being.

Believe it or not, small talk has been the subject of considerable academic research over the years. According to Australian academic and researcher Dr. Justine Coupland who has studied the phenomenon of small talk in depth, small talk fulfils our human need to be connected to others socially. It's not a substantive, philosophical examination of your existential angst. But it does reflect your thought processes and, even if you don't intend it to, it become the basis for both you and others to draw conclusions.

It's crucially important to both your health – mental, physical and emotional – and to the health care that will assist you in achieving maximum good health that you think carefully about how you describe your well-being…even if it seems like so much small talk. Your common sense will tell you that responding, "I'm really well," will have a different impact both on others and on you personally than if you respond, "So-so." It may be the case that whenever you ask someone how he or she is, you don't really want to know. That being said, how that person responds does have an impact on what you think about them and their situation, and how the conversation progresses. It's exactly the same in your own head. Remember that what is perceived as real is real in all its consequences.

There used to be a saying that is very likely familiar to you: "Sticks and stones may break my bones, but names (or words) will never hurt me…" It's time you were seriously disabused of that idea. Names, labels, words   all of these have a significant ability to hurt you, or make you better. And when it comes to mindless chatter, that's perhaps even a more significant issue for you and your health.

I'm talking about the kind of mind-dump where you say – either out loud to others or to just yourself – everything that comes into your mind. These words surface mindlessly without any consideration of the effects they may have on the listeners – whether the listener is you or other people. This is even more significant today where this kind of mind-dumping can be broadcast to the world to huge audiences via social media. And people from the most obscure to the most powerful individuals in our society are prone to this kind of reckless verbal carnage. It's important the you're not one of them if you intend to live well until you die.

EXAMINING YOUR OWN VOCABULARY

Have you ever really taken the time to consider your own vocabulary? Your vocabulary is the body of words that you use most often. It's likely that you've never given this much thought since your words have evolved over the course of your life. They are simply how you communicate verbally.

You learned certain words from your family (the words your family used for specific body parts, for example), but your vocabulary has also been, and continues to be, influenced by other factors. Your education, what and how much you read, the films and television you watch – all of these are important factors. However, one of the most insidious contributors to your vocabulary is the social interactions you have in person, and increasingly, online. And the truth is that words can come to mean more or less by their usage.

The word "awesome", for example, is one that used to be applied to things such as the experience of seeing the Grand Canyon or Michelangelo's *David* for the first time. But it hardly seems an appropriate descriptor in these situations any longer when everything from the cup of coffee you had this morning, to the YouTube video you just watched is described that way. If you habitually refer to everything as awesome or perfect, then nothing is really awesome or perfect. Those words become meaningless. That being said, your word choice when referring to yourself can affect your health and well-being in ways you probably could never imagine.

Freud once said, "Words have a magical power. They can either bring the greatest happiness or the deepest despair." It is worth your while to consider his meaning as we explore the concept of your ***personal dictionary.***

Your personal dictionary consists of all the words and phrases and their meanings – that you habitually use in conversation with yourself and others.

A personal dictionary is fundamental. Most of us are unaware that we have such a dictionary within us. Our use of certain terms is symptomatic of how we are thinking about the underlying issues, and when we are communicating about our health, we often use our own dictionaries instead of our common sense when we interpret what others, including healthcare providers, are saying to us.

It's not just a question of positive words versus negative ones. That's too simplistic. Try not to think of words that way, despite what all the pop psychology gurus say. Your words are neither positive, nor are they negative...but their effects can be to enhance your life or to detract from your health and life.

Sit down and make a list of the words that you generally use to describe yourself to others. What do you say when someone asks you how you are? What do you say to your friends and family about the state of your physical, mental or emotional health? What words do you use more often than others in general conversation? You are beginning to get a picture of your personal dictionary. Now you need to consider each of the words and reflect on how each one makes you feel. Is there a better word.? Are there words that you would like to be able to apply to yourself? Write those down as well.

The next step is to think about how your words might be affecting others. What conclusions might others draw about you based simply on those words? Remember that the conclusions they draw will have a direct impact on how they treat you. Are these the outcomes that make you feel better? Common sense tells you that if you have control over how others respond to you, it is in your best interests to make that response one that serves you well. You need to create a personal dictionary that works for you rather than against you.

Words are a major part of your conversations with yourself and others, but they are not the only part.

THE CONCEPT OF FRAMING...AND REFRAMING

The words you choose mindfully are only the start. Whether you recognize it or not, you then put those words within a frame.

> **A frame is the boundary within which you create a story.**

Your frame is made up of the parameters you choose. You might even call this the spin, to use a media term. It is, for example, the way you choose to show only a small part of your life in your Facebook or Instagram feed, or how you choose to tell a story to your friends or family, or even how you choose to tell a story to yourself.

The Hugh Jackman film *The Greatest Showman* is a good illustration of what I mean by framing. It's the story of PT Barnum of Barnum and Bailey circus fame (among many other things that we hear less about). PT Barnum has gone down in history mostly as the master of the publicity having been widely quoted as having said, "There's a sucker born every minute," but no one really knows for sure if he said it. In any case, that's how we have most often seen his story framed.

This film tells the same story – hyperbolic promotion, hiring the outcasts of society and exploiting them – but it does it within a totally different frame than we might be used to. In this version of his story, it's about his humanity: how he offered these people a living, a home, acceptance and ultimately the family they never had. Same story – told from a very different perspective – framed differently.

... if thought corrupts language, language can also corrupt thought. ~ George Orwell

Framing alters your perception of the world. What elements of a story you see or hear, and what is left out, what is emphasized, and what is down played, are key to your understanding of that narrative. Consider the words you use to describe your complaint when you are sitting in your doctor's examining room. Then consider what you have selected to leave out, as well as what you have decided to emphasize. This is your frame. Your doctor is limited in his or her ability to truly understand you because of that frame which may or may not permit full disclosure of your problem. This can seriously hamper your healthcare provider from doing his or her job optimally.

There is another area of your life when understanding framing might just be the most common sense tool you have to get the most for your life and health. If you understand the concept of framing, and think about it whenever you are exposed to advertising or the promotion of health-related ideas or products (regardless of whether that promotion is coming from a drug company, celebrity or any other source), you should consider the slant of the promotion.

INTERPRETING A FRAME

- **What words are being used?**
- **What slant or spin is being applied?**
- **What is being left out?**
- **What is being emphasized?**
- **What is being down-played?**
- **Who benefits from you reacting positively to the message?**

Answering all of these questions will help you to figure out what is really being said and what you are being persuaded to do. But more than that, you will begin to see how you are often manipulated into a particular conclusion simply because you don't have a broader frame within which to interpret the message. The more often you do this, the easier it becomes.

THE DANGER OF EUPHEMISMS

How often do you hear one person telling another that someone has "passed away" or, even worse, "passed"? Perhaps you use these terms yourself. There is nothing fundamentally wrong with saying that someone who has actually died has "passed away" (although it is not as clear), but the habit of using such terminology can be problematic for you if what you're really trying to do is get the most out of your life and healthcare. What you are doing is using euphemistic language, and that can be dangerous for you.

> *Euphemism is a human device to conceal the horrors of reality.* ~ Paul Johnson

A euphemism is often described as a polite way of saying something that might otherwise be interpreted as too harsh, or even too real.

> **A euphemism can be defined as a word or phrase that is substituted for another – usually more precise one – that is used in place of an uncomfortable one.**

Euphemistic terms are often used innocuously, but they can be problematic if they represent an unwillingness to confront the reality represented by the more "correct" word.

Governments often use the term "collateral damage" for example when they really mean women and children killed during a war strike that wasn't actually targeted at them. There are many such terms that politicians use, and we generally realize what they mean, although the precise meaning is often obscured leading to the distinct possibility of misinterpretation. Even more problematic than those, however, are the euphemistic terms that you may use to describe aspects of your own life and health. Many such terms permit you to avoid truly seeing the issue for what it is. If you cannot see an issue honestly and for what it truly means to you, you cannot deal with it.

These euphemisms are often ambiguous thus don't really serve you well if you use them to communicate with others – or even with yourself. When talking to yourself, euphemisms are nothing short of lying: in polite society they might well be thought of as kind, but this is a social convention. Talking to yourself is different.

Here are some of the most widely used and least helpful euphemistic terms that you may find yourself using.

Euphemism you may be using	The more precise, realistic term
passed away, passed, passed on	died
the big "C"	cancer
chemical dependency	drug addiction
big boned, husky, curvy, full-figured	overweight, fat
offed him/herself	committed suicide
aurally challenged, hearing impaired	deaf
mentally challenged	mentally ill
adult beverages	liquor

Although many euphemisms that we use in day-to-day life are not terribly problematic, there are some health-related ones you may find yourself using that can indicate you may not be facing the reality of the situation.

At this point you may be asking why it is, then that it seems the medical community itself uses euphemisms. The kind of communication used in medical circles is less euphemistic than it is professional jargon. The fact is that jargon, in whatever industry, becomes the way that members of that industry can understand one another and communicate precisely. That does not mean that it is acceptable for your family physician, for example, to use the medical community's jargon when communicating with you, the patient.

For example, when you are preparing for surgery and your doctor tells you that you have to be "NPO" after midnight, you should not be expected to understand this without further explanation. If he or she says that to the nurse who is looking after you in the hospital, that is perfectly acceptable since the nurse, a fellow healthcare worker, will know that this means that you are to have "nothing by mouth" (it is an acronym for the Latin phrase *nil per os*), and that will then be conveyed to you in terms you understand.

In the same vein, members of the medical community often use words or phrases that could be better chosen. They don't always consider the effect their words may have when you, the patient, then turn around and use the same words to describe yourself.

One such phrase that is too often used to describe more or less successful treatment of chronic diseases such as cancer is "in remission" as in, "Your cancer is in remission." You are now supposed to be happy about this. Put yourself in this position for a moment and think about what this would mean to you and how you live your life.

When a medical condition is "in remission" it actually means that the signs and symptoms of the disease have disappeared following some kind of treatment. In order for the medical community to consider you "cured" you have to be "in remission" for an almost arbitrarily-determined length of time, depending on your condition. I say arbitrary because even that could be wrong. When they refer to your condition as "in complete remission" with no detectable aspects of the disease whatsoever, they are still not willing to say you are "cured." Some of this is a result of the fact that doctors prefer not to be sued by unnecessarily litigious patients. What's a patient to do, then?

The truth is that you are potentially "cured." Isn't that a very different way to think about yourself and your disease than to be always thinking that it might return any moment? Common sense suggests that if worrying about the potential return of a disease overshadows your ability to live your life as a healthy person, you are better served to consider yourself at least potentially cured. You're only ever healthy until you aren't. Your glass should always be half full.

APPLYING COMMON SENSE TO YOUR VOCABULARY CHOICES

How do you define yourself in terms of your health? Healthy? Sick? Okay? Victim? Survivor? The words you use to define yourself are very telling about how you feel about yourself. However, even more important perhaps is that they are going to be predictive of your health outcomes.

Here are the words that I consider to be the most dangerous words you can apply to yourself in relation to your health:

- **Victim**
- **Hero**
- **Survivor**
- **Fearful**
- **Worried**
- **Anxious**
- **Stupid**
- **Brave**

I am fairly certain that you often hear these words in relation to people with health concerns. I am also convinced that you (and others) consider more than one of them to be positive. From my point of view, these words are all equally dangerous to you when trying to apply common sense to thinking about your own health.

Let's look at the word *survivor* first. Describing people who have dealt with a cancer diagnosis (and are still alive) as survivors on an ongoing basis says several (unhealthy) things. First, the word survivor means a person who continues to live after facing death. Sound okay to you? Here's why it should raise red flags. If you have "survived" cancer, and you continue to think of yourself as a "survivor" you are never far away from those thoughts that you could have died – and could die. Of course, you *are* going to die: life is, after all, terminal for everyone. However, making that a daily part of how you think about yourself prevents you from simply carrying on living.

The word *victim* is perhaps even more dangerous. What is a victim? A victim is someone who has been attacked, harmed, injured or killed – someone who has been damaged by some kind of unpleasant event. Although, on the face of it, you might well consider yourself to be a victim of something – cancer victim or sexual assault victim to name two of the most ubiquitous – but consider this: do you always want to think of yourself as someone who has been damaged? Or would you like to live the rest of your life considering yourself to be a healthy human being who has put a negative experience in his or her past? A common sense approach to making the best of the life you have left suggests that you need to first stop thinking of yourself as a victim, then impress upon those who are in your personal circle that you have stopped thinking about yourself in those terms.   Remember this: *Refer to yourself as a victim – whether speaking or thinking – and you risk losing any semblance of personal control; you are giving control of your life to the illness or aggressor.* The first step in taking control is to stop thinking about yourself as a victim.

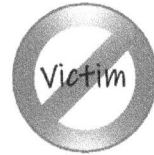

All the other words on this list are similar in terms of how they make you feel in the long term. The label *hero* is an interesting one. A hero is someone who is idealized for his or her bravery, courage or achievements. If you are looked upon as a hero by your friends and family simply because you handled your difficult diagnosis with dignity, you will always be in that kind of idealized frame. The only way you can continue to be a hero is for the situation that made you a hero continue. In other words, you will always be a hero if you are always thought of in terms of your particular illness. It would be healthier for you to get out of that frame and into a life where you can be treated like a normal, healthy individual. Your experience will always be with you, but it does not have to define who you are as you live the rest of your life.

It's worth considering learning to picture illness as *a part* of you, rather than as something separate from you that you have to deal with – or worse, fight against. First accept it as a part of you and work with it. Consider what it means or does not mean to you. Recognizing your cancer or arthritis, for example, as a part of you (which it is) does not mean, however, that it *is* you – it does not need to define you. You only need to recognize it as a part of who you are. What you continually resist in yourself will insist on making its way into your life one way or another.

There is a whole other set of words that are problematic for you if you are in the middle of dealing with an illness, and they are all a part of a paradigm – a certain way that medical treatment is framed. Those words relate to thinking of medical treatment as war.

Here are some dangerous words that are often applied to illness treatment.

- **Battle**
- **War**
- **Fight**

All of these words signify a very dangerous idea: that your illness is something outside of you that you have to fight. Since it is really a part of you, all you end up doing is fighting against yourself. The outcome can never be as healthy as it should be.

Argue for your limitations, and sure enough they're yours. ~ Richard Bach

If treatment for a disease is seen as a *war* in which you have to *fight* battles, the outcome is either that you *win* or you *lose*. Does that mean that if the treatment does not achieve the planned objective that you have lost? If you have lost the battle and the war, then what's keeping you alive? We, as a society, need to stop thinking about disease treatment as a war – and we need to stop fighting. Even if your treatment does not achieve the objectives it was intended to, that does not mean that you have lost. You simply have to face a new reality. The bottom line in all of this is to select your vocabulary carefully, and face the reality with a certain degree of optimism.

We tend to be a bit OC (obsessive-compulsive) when we're using words to describe our relationship with our health. OC is like shining a spotlight: you see only where the light points. If you change the focal point to another area or blur the initial one or the background out, you can change how you think and feel about yourself. Your words = your perception. Personal perceptions give rise to our emotions.

Yehuda Berg, author of the best-selling book *The Power of Kabbalah* once wrote:

> *"Words are singularly the most powerful force available to humanity. We can choose to use this force constructively with words of encouragement, or destructively using words of despair. Words have energy and power with the ability to help, to heal, to hinder, to hurt, to harm, to humiliate and to humble."*

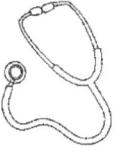

KEYS TO IMPROVING YOUR USE OF WORDS

☑ Avoid mindless, knee-jerk responses to others and to yourself.

☑ Listen to yourself then consciously use words that have a positive effect on your well-being.

☑ Be mindful of the words you choose to describe yourself; be clear about the outcomes you'd like to achieve.

☑ Carefully select the words you use when interacting with health professionals.

☑ Avoid euphemistic language in favour of realistic terminology.

☑ Focus on dealing with reality.

☑ Stop seeing the medical treatment of disease as some kind of war.

☑ Stop fighting.

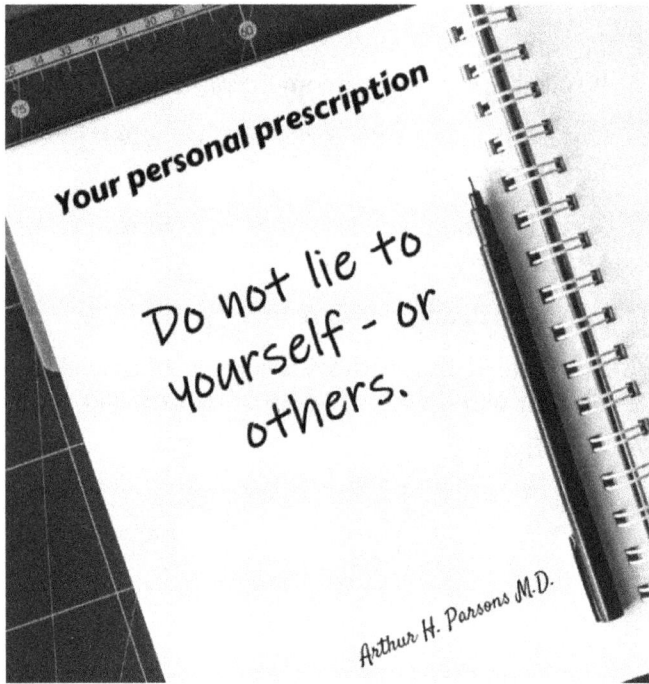

CHAPTER SIX

BE CAREFUL WHO YOU LISTEN TO: THE PERILS OF OUTSIDE INFLUENCE

"It is the mark of an educated mind to be able to entertain a thought without accepting it." ~Aristotle

IN A RECENT AMERICAN STUDY of where consumers obtain most of their health information, researchers found that the majority of people seek and find the bulk of their health information from mass media, far outstripping the number of people whose primary source of information is a health professional. This has been the case for some time now. In addition, almost a third of the searches that are done today on the World Wide Web are on health-related topics. (80% of Internet users have searched online for health information at some point, up from 62% in 2001). The sad truth is that the research also discovered that there is a continuing and accelerating problem with the quality of the information found online. It is often sub-standard. But that's not the only place where you will find sub-standard health and life advice.

Consider that other popular source of information: the solicited, or often even unsolicited, guidance that you're likely to receive from your mother, sister, friend (real and imagined), co-worker or pharmaceutical company, to mention a few. The problem is trying to figure out whose information is truly accurate, beneficial material and whose information is bogus. A big dose of common sense would go a long way here, but when people are vulnerable, as those seeking health advice often are, common sense seems to be fleeting at best. It's time to learn to use your own common sense (with a few outside tips) to analyse critically the information that bombards you from all angles. It may even be the case that your well-meaning (but usually self-serving) best friend might have to be ignored.

THE PERILS OF LISTENING TO "MEDIA INFLUENCERS"

You know the people I'm talking about. Dr. Oz, Oprah, Gwyneth Paltrow, the Kardashians, Jenny McCarthy, popular YouTubers and the list goes on. These individuals are people who have become celebrities by way of their media exposure not because they have any education, knowledge or expertise in anything remotely health-related – with the exception of Dr. Oz who is in a separate, if overlapping category. (I'll get back to Dr. Oz later in this chapter.) Sometimes these people use professionals with that important expertise to support their advice, and sometimes it's accurate and worthwhile. In these cases, the "celebrity" is only the face of the issue whereas the medical professional is the real source. However, more often than not, it is well worth your while to use a bit of common sense when listening to them. And yet, many people listen to them without even a modicum of critical analysis – or even common sense. Here's an example.

A few years ago, Gwyneth Paltrow, by way of her website *Goop*, gave this advice: steam your vagina. Not even an abundance of common sense was needed here to come to the conclusion that any woman steaming her vagina in response to an actor's advice was, at least a sucker, or at worst, clearly doing her body a disservice. If something sounds wrong, it probably is. Here is what she said:

"You sit on what is essentially a mini-throne, and a combination of infrared and mugwort steam cleanses your uterus, et al. It is an energetic release – not just a steam douche – that balances female hormone levels. If you're in LA, you have to do it."

First, even a modicum of anatomical understanding (which I hope every adult woman has) indicates clearly that steam entering via your vagina will not reach inside your uterus. Second, your uterus is definitely not in need of steaming, and the temperature of real steam is above 100 degrees

It has been suggested that human beings are evolutionarily wired to follow and, perhaps, be influenced by people they look up to. ~ Dr. Timothy Caulfield

Celsius (212 degrees Fahrenheit), high enough to burn you in areas where you do not want to be burned. Third, how in the world can anyone make a connection between externally applied steam and hormone levels?

And Paltrow, via her *Goop* seems to be in love, generally, with the concept of internal cleansing. There is no scientific evidence that any of Paltrow's so-called cleansing of internal organs is necessary or beneficial, and in some cases it can actually be harmful. And yet...

In 2016 Dr. Timothy Caulfield, Research Director of the University of Alberta's Health Law Institute, wrote a book titled: *Is Gwyneth Paltrow Wrong About Everything? When Celebrity Culture and Science Clash*. The book explores celebrity health and wellness claims (he even visited the *Goop* offices to try to find out about their cleanse), the science (or mostly lack thereof) behind it, and why people are prone to following such nonsensical advice. Oh, the short answer to the question he posed in the book's title: yes.

After celebrities, there are the online influencers who are, in themselves, usually not true celebrities, but their thousands of

YouTube or Instagram followers tell a different story. And these people have become the darlings of product and service marketers. In fact, there is a new marketing approach called *influencer marketing*.

According to the *Huffington Post* in 2016, influencer marketing is defined as: "...the action of promoting and selling products or services through people (influencers) who have the capacity to have an effect on the character of a brand." This isn't new. It is really a twenty-first century riff on third-party endorsement. The company seeks out someone else – someone outside the organization who appeals to or is known by the members of the target market – to sell you on the product. These days, instead of creating ad *copy*, they create a *narrative* to tell you a story you can identify with, because you are the target. And the person telling you that story will be someone you follow on social media and whose stories are likely to go viral. And why does this person do this? Does this influencer deeply believe in the product? Maybe, but the real underlying reason this influencer will act like that old-time snake-oil salesman is because he or she is being *paid* to do so. So, buyer beware.

This is how you are manipulated by influencers:

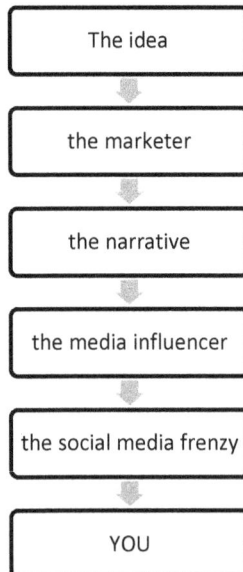

The idea

↓

the marketer

↓

the narrative

↓

the media influencer

↓

the social media frenzy

↓

YOU

One sub-category of influencers are those health professionals with credentials. These may be some of the most problematic. I promised I'd get back to Dr. Oz, and here is the category into which he falls. Although he is a credentialed surgeon, you are no doubt aware his peers in the medical profession have been trying to censure him for many of the products and services he has promoted over the years since they lack scientific support, or evidence of any kind short of the vague anecdotes from people who swear by them (refer back to Chapter 3, "The Placebo Effect"). In 2014 he even received a "scolding" from a congressional committee after which he promised to do better "fact-checking." According to a 2017 piece in the *American Medical Association Journal of Ethics*, "Ten physicians wrote to the medical school dean at Columbia [where he holds a faculty position] claiming that he was endangering public health, had demonstrated contempt for medical and scientific evidence, and was ineligible to sit on the faculty of a prestigious medical institution."

Over the years he has told mothers that there were high doses of arsenic in their children's apples when the evidence indicated that this was

> *A lie repeated often enough becomes the truth.* ~ G. Goebbles

false; he has told his viewing audience on more than one occasion that genetically modified foods definitely cause cancer when there is no evidence to support this claim; he promoted green bean coffee as a sure-fire weight-loss solution – it is not… and the list goes on.

The most egregious problem that you face when confronted with so-called experts like Dr. Oz is that he does have those credentials, and ought to know better. However, you also need to keep in mind that since he was "discovered" by Oprah, he has become a media star much more than he has stayed a medical expert – in cardiovascular surgery, I must point out despite the fact that he seems to have knowledge of every specialty out there.

If it seems that no individual doctor could possibly know that much about so many disparate specialties, common sense tells you that he doesn't. Then it's just a matter of ensuring that you listen to your common sense.

How pseudoscience is infiltrating the online influencers

One of the most insidious problems that you have as a health consumer trying to make the best decisions for getting through life is trying to figure out if the information you see or hear is based on real science or pseudoscience. It wasn't always this hard, but pseudoscience has become a growing problem in recent years. Here's how I define it:

Pseudoscience is any activity or evidence that purports to be based on science or resembles science, but is based on deceptive assumptions, lacks supporting evidence or reasonableness, and cannot be reliably tested.

In short, pseudoscience is false science that stretches the limits of common sense. How can you tell when something you are seeing is an example of pseudoscience? Here are some of the characteristics that indicate what you're seeing might not be what it appears.

The following chart identifies the major characteristics of something that is masquerading as science but does not stand up to real scrutiny. (Before you read this, you might consider re-reading the section in Chapter Four: "What makes something science.")

The idea is dogmatic.	A dogmatic position or belief is one that is deemed by its proponents o be accepted as authority. As such, it is not to be disputed or doubted.
The idea is aimed directly at the public.	It seems to have been created just for you without benefit of peer review.
It is conveyed by verbose language and lots of jargon.	The use of so many words seems to be designed to confuse you.
The claims appear vague and/or untestable.	If no one else has tested it, it might not be true. If it is ambiguous, unclear, or otherwise vague, it is suspect.
It exhibits "confirmational bias."	This means that the evidence presented has been carefully selected to cover up any information that might dispute the claims being made.
It presents anecdotes as evidence.	Refer back to Chapter Four.
The narrative about it suggests that it cannot be tested scientifically.	Need I say more?
There are no clear explanations of how the product, service of activity actually works.	Vaginal steaming, anyone?

Regardless of the credentials of the person babbling on about scientific issues in the media, if the narrative is riddled with any number of these characteristics, your common sense needs to kick in: remain just a bit, if not a lot, sceptical.

Carl Sagan once wrote: "I maintain there is much more wonder in science than in pseudoscience. And in addition, to whatever measure this term has any meaning, science has the additional virtue, and it is not an inconsiderable one, of being true." There may be virtue in the truth.

WHY LISTENING TO YOUR FAMILY OR "FRIENDS" MAY NOT BE THE BEST STRATEGY

How do we define a friend these days? Every dictionary available to us suggests that a friend has the following characteristics:

- Someone you know;

- Someone with whom you have some kind of a bond, like mutual affection;

- Someone on whom you could count if you ever need help;

- Someone who is happy to spend time with you;

- Someone with whom you share mutual trust;

- Someone who is on your side.

If these are the criteria for defining someone as a friend, then I suggest that most of us have very few real friends. Many of us have lots of acquaintances, and even more contacts through social media, some of whom you might call a "friend" if you're talking about at least one specific platform (*Facebook*, anyone?). But for the purposes of this discussion of determining whether or not to listen to your friends when it comes to health-related and life advice, I would include them all. And family members also suffer from the same issues.

Consider the following situation. A young mother decides that she is prepared to listen to a celebrity's anti-vaccination propaganda, and chooses to avoid vaccinating her baby against the advice of her family physician. Then, instead of simply keeping this to herself, the next time she meets her friends who share play dates with her and her child, she asks the other mothers if they are planning to have their children vaccinated. When her best friend indicates to her that she has set up the appointment with her doctor, the first young mother begins her attempt to convince her friend that she should avoid these vaccinations. This line of conversation repeats itself every time the two mothers meet over the next six months. The more the second mother "sticks to her guns," the more the first mother "doubles down" on her efforts to convince her friend. Even after the second mother has had her baby vaccinated, the first mother continues to suggest that she will regret it. Should the second mother have followed her friend's advice?

The issue here is one that I have seen over and over in my medical practice, and in my private life. A patient has a friend or family member who is attempting, with every argument at his or her disposal, to convince others to follow their lead. What I have observed is that this is less a situation of real, heart-felt concern for others than it is an attempt on the part of someone to rally others to their cause, thereby further supporting their contention that their own decision was the right one. If others are taking a different route, this puts their decision into questionable territory. And it happens all the time. Your friends want you to do what they do. If they convince you to follow their lead, they are able to reinforce their own decisions. If you don't, as in the case of the anti-vaccination mother in the story, your friends will double down on their attempts to get you to follow. Be prepared. I have seen many patients who have problems dealing with this doubling down. They have dealt with this by finally agreeing to follow the recommendations (or demands) of the other person, yet doing what they wanted to in the first place. In effect, they choose to lie.

Apart from the fact that your friends and family are not experts in most of the advice they bestow upon you, their motives for offering it to you in the first place are suspect. "But my friends and family only have my best interests at heart," you might protest. When you think deeply about this, and apply some common sense to the process, you will soon begin to agree with me that this is usually bulls**t. Those people might very well think highly of you and your well-being, but their prime motivator in the specific situation is usually themselves – not you. It's important not to be sucked in when someone is telling you something that you believe not to be entirely right for you.

Even more egregious is the problem with online "friends." It's important to come right out with it at the outset when discussing this category of purveyors of unwelcome advice. They do not have YOUR BEST INTERESTS AT HEART. You do not share a BOND OF MUTUAL AFFECTION. You have no basis upon which to TRUST them. They are not ON YOUR SIDE. So, it is nonsensical to follow their advice. You need other sources of information.

So, if you are no longer going to put blind faith into friends, family and social media, what's left? What about health professionals? Are they always right? Not always.

BEING AWARE OF THE PITFALLS OF PROFESSIONAL PEOPLE AND GROUPS

BEWARE OF PATIENT ADVOCACY GROUPS

You've just been diagnosed with irritable bowel syndrome. You decide to search online to see if you can find help from others in the same situation. During this online research, you discover that there are several relevant patient advocacy groups. They all seem to offer the kind of support and advice you need so you decide to become a member of one. Over time, as you participate in their online forums and discussions, and read their blogs, most of the other patients seem to be taking a particular medication. On your next visit to your physician, you tell her that you would like to be put on this new medication. When your doctor demurs, indicating to you that in her opinion your current medication regime is the right one for you, what do you do? Are you aware that you have been following the advice of a patient advocacy group that receives a large proportion of its funding from the pharmaceutical company that produces the drug you are requesting? Are you aware that the prime motivator for the drug company's financial support of this group is actually to sell their drugs? If you don't, and this understanding has never played a part in your evaluation of the advice you're receiving from an organization that seems to consist of your peers, you are not alone. But it's time you took a closer look. Perhaps it's time you listened to your common sense and did some due diligence.

Over the past decade there have been increasing numbers of studies focused on the relationship between drug companies and patient support groups. In one study published in in 2017 in the *New England Journal of Medicine* (arguably one of the most influential medical journals in the world), American researchers studied 107 of the largest of these groups in the US – including such organizations as the American Heart Association, American Liver Foundation, American Kidney Foundation, Autism Speaks, the Arthritis Foundation, the Alliance for Lupus Research, the Epilepsy Foundation, the National Multiple Sclerosis Society, the Leukaemia and Lymphoma Society, the March of Dimes, the Prostate Cancer Foundation and the list goes on. (The study is listed in the sources at the end of this book and is linked to a complete list.). What they discovered is fascinating – and an eye-opener for many patients.

They found that 36% of the organizations had at least one board member representing the drug, device or biotechnology industry, and a large proportion of those held leadership positions on the board. However, a quarter of the organizations (26% to be precise) disclosed no information on the current or past employment of its board members. In addition – and this is where you need to pay attention – 83% of these organizations reported receiving financial support from industry, and of the remaining 17%, most published no information on their financial support. A large proportion of the funding was in amounts over $1 million a year.

Another example: In early 2018 American Senator Claire McCaskill released another example of research tying patient advocacy groups to big pharma. Her study found that in the five years between 2012 and 2017, five of the leading opioid manufacturers in the U.S. had contributed a whopping $9 million to patient advocacy groups, and what was more disturbing, the research found that, in fact, this had exerted influence over the activities of the groups. And there are countless other studies that support the same conclusions.

Then consider the fact that events like Breast Cancer Awareness month have similarly dubious histories. This awareness month was created in 1985 as a public relations strategy for what was then Imperial Chemical Industries (now AstraZeneca which is a major producer of breast cancer drugs) as a partnership between them and the American Cancer Society. Imperial Chemical Industries, by the way, was a manufacturer of a variety of chemical products including paints, artificial flavourings and chemical fertilizers. If this feels a bit odd to you, you might be remembering that there have been links between chemical fertilizer exposure and – breast cancer. (For an eye-opening exposure of the breast cancer industry, consider watching the National Film Board of Canada's documentary film *Pink Ribbons Inc.*) This kind of PR approach is what is referred to as cause-related marketing, with an emphasis on the marketing – of whatever the company produces. This awareness often changes how people feel about these kinds of schemes.

It's difficult in these days of so-called "fake news" to ferret out the truth from the hype in many aspects of our lives. It is especially important, though, to try when it comes to your health. Common sense suggests that it's important for you to look deeper. If you're happy with the over-riding motivation behind the advice, then it is your absolute choice to follow it. However, blindly accepting such advice is reckless.

So, at least you can count on your doctor? Well, usually.

KNOW YOUR OWN DOCTOR

After 45 years in medical practice, I can tell you without a doubt that pharmaceutical companies influence many doctors' prescribing habits. But do you know if your doctor is one of them?

It was a regular occurrence in my large medical practice. Like clockwork, every couple of days, the drug reps would arrive (with a prior appointment, of course) and set up a display so that during the day the various family physicians and specialists who regularly held office hours in our clinic would wander by for a look and a discussion. Naturally, if you ask a drug rep the purpose of these displays, you will be told that it is to *educate* the doctors about the newest and shiniest

> *Doubt everything or believe everything: these are two equally convenient strategies. With either we dispense with the need for reflection.*
> ~ Henri Poincare

pharmaceutical marvel. It is true that there are so many new drugs popping up (many of which are significantly more expensive than the older products) that any information that helps with the prescribing could be useful. However, that's not the whole story.

The real objective of these drug reps is to persuade/ convince/ encourage/ induce more doctors to use their product over any similar product offered by their competitors. Over the years, doctors have generally held the opinion that their prescribing habits are not unduly influenced by the marketing strategies of drug companies, but my own personal experience as well as studies examining physician prescribing habits have told a different story.

It seems that the pharmaceutical industry thinks that influencing physician prescribing habits is important and successful enough that it spends almost $90 billion a year worldwide on drug rep – doctor interactions which accounted for 60% of their marketing budgets. A study published in the *British Medical Journal* in 2017 drew the following conclusion:

*"...Physician–pharmaceutical industry and its sales
representatives' interactions and acceptance of gifts from the
company's PSRs have been found to affect physicians'
prescribing behaviour and are likely to contribute to irrational
prescribing of the company's drug..."*

Does this mean that your doctor may have been influenced
to prescribe a particular drug for you? Maybe.

In the early years of my medical career I would interact with
these drug sales people, but in the last 30 years, I avoided them at
all costs. The only reason they were even in the office on a regular
basis was that I shared a large practice with 17 other family
physicians and not all of them held the same opinion of the drug
companies that I did. Should you ask your doctor about his or her
dealings with drug companies? It would make good sense to do
so if you are questioning his or her prescribing habits.

However, influence by drug companies is not always so
direct as the drug rep-doctor interaction. Doctors are also
indirectly influenced by industry via what is known in the
medical community as the *consensus group*.

A consensus group is a group of qualified specialists
brought together under the auspices of a variety of umbrella
organizations most of which are heavily funded by the
pharmaceutical industry. When consensus groups first began in
the 1970's, they were a good idea: a group of well-qualified
specialists brought together by government agencies to discuss
the current state of affairs within a particular topic area. They
were not designed to provide treatment guidelines. However, as
big pharma became more involved, many devolved into meetings
where the invited specialists are housed in elegant hotels, fed
lavish meals and entertained (this includes their spouse/
significant other in many instances) while they meet during the
day to review treatment guidelines for specific medical concerns.
For example, they might be meeting to discuss best practices in
the treatment of high blood pressure.

At the beginning of the meeting they will review current guidelines that might, for instance, suggest that hypertension is defined as anyone with a blood pressure over 140/90. After some discussion, the group might come to a consensus that blood pressures over 120/80 ought to be treated, thereby effectively instantly increasing the potential market share for the company or companies who are footing the bill for the meeting: a pharmaceutical company that makes anti-hypertensive medications. This guideline for treatment then becomes gospel even though the science is not behind it may not be conclusive or even evident at all. If you research the members of any individual consensus group, you will find that many of the participants, at some point in their career, had some kind of cooperative dealing with a drug company that produces these very drugs needed to treat the disease. Often, at some point in the past they have been paid by the drug companies as expert speakers, or their research

The great enemy of the truth is very often not the lie - deliberate, contrived, and dishonest - but the myth - persistent, persuasive, and unrealistic. ~ John F. Kennedy

has been supported, in part, by a grant from big pharma.

What this means to you is that if your current drug regimen is working for you, it's imperative that you question a change in medication or overall approach. Be sure you ask your doctor to explain "why" you need this new approach.

FINALLY: FOLLOW THE MONEY

It may already be self-evident to you that there seems to be a recurring theme throughout this chapter. Apart from our discussion of being aware of following advice from your friends, all of the rest seems to suggest that you need to look closely at one thing: the money.

Who has paid that media influencer you listen to? Whose pocket is your doctor in, if anybody's? Have your friends spent money on stuff they now want you to adopt? Are they somehow emotionally attached to the decision they have made? It so often traces back to money as the prime motivator. When you're trying to figure out the best source for health and life information, it's clear that when money is in the mix, it muddies the water making it much more difficult for you to know when your best interests are at the heart of it.

Here are some questions to consider when trying to figure this out. Answer these questions to follow the money.

Who benefits most from you following the advice?
If the answer is not you, then consider if this works for you in spite of it.

What advice is being offered?
Is it really advice that is specifically tailored to the situation?

When was this information written/created/reviewed last?
Is it up to date?

Where did the information come from?
Is the source a knowledgeable expert? A celebrity? A non-medical friend? Can you trust this source?

Why is this source providing this advice?
Is this source simply trying to get you to support his or her decision/product/idea?

And back to the top: Is the fact that the source is making money from your adoption of the advice outweighing their concern for your life and health? The final piece of advice above takes us right back to the beginning: *caveat emptor*...buyer beware. And always remember to follow the money.

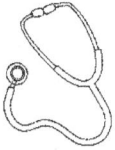

KEYS TO KNOWING WHO TO LISTEN TO

☑ Be sure that the person (or group) you are listening to has the knowledge and expertise to provide accurate information.

☑ If you think the claims are too good to be true, you're probably right.

☑ Check to be sure that the information is current.

☑ Remember that just because you trust someone as a friend does not mean that you should trust that person when he or she gives you medical or health-related information. It is only their opinion.

☑ Always be sure you are well aware of who benefits from you buying or buying into this health-related information or product.

☑ Maintain a healthy skepticism when anyone – whether your friend, your mother or a favourite celebrity – tries to convince you to take action related to your health.

☑ Follow the money.

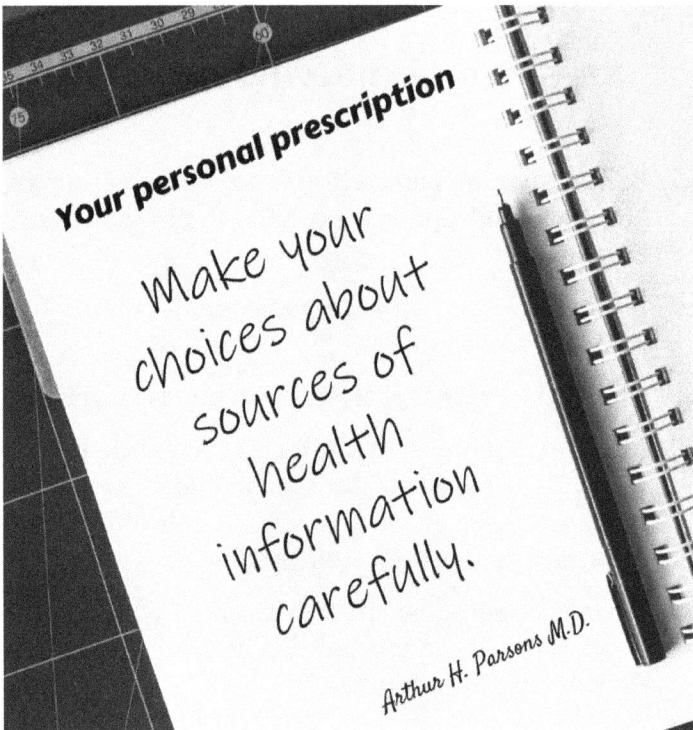

Your personal prescription

Make your choices about sources of health information carefully.

Arthur H. Parsons M.D.

CHAPTER SEVEN

IF LIFE IS TERMINAL, DO I STILL NEED (HEALTH) GOALS? YES!

"A journey of a thousand miles begins with a single step."
~ Lao-Tzu

LIFE IS CERTAINLY A JOURNEY – one in which you know that there is an end point, but you have no idea when you'll reach it. I've often thought that it's a good thing we don't know. However, it does mean that we need to consider how we want to live each day – just in case it's our last. But if it is the journey rather than the endpoint that's important, do you still need to have goals? In my view, the answer is yes.

As we begin our discussion of the kinds of goals that are helpful in moving toward that terminus at the end of your life (and doing it well), it's important to begin with a firm understanding of the fact that life is non-negotiable, but living that life – *how* you do it – definitely *is*. This is where those goals begin to make sense for you.

Goal-setting is a skill that many people lack. This is the reason that so many life coaches have popped up like weeds sprouting in the spring. There is a whole industry devoted to helping you learn to set goals to achieve all manner of "success." But there always seems to be an assumption that success is generally concrete (money or fame, for example) and that it is the real end game. The kind of goal setting we'll explore together is focused more on achieving those on-going intentions that signify to you that you are living your best life, regardless of your wealth or health status. Let's take a common sense exploration of the land through which you are journeying.

THE FORGOTTEN LAND OF HEALTH

It's fairly safe to say that whenever the terms "health" or "health care" are being discussed, the real focus is illness or what I like to call "dis-ease." How can I avoid *illness*? How can I deal with *illness*? Even people heavily invested in industries that purport to be health conscious – the booming nutrition supplement industry for example – are largely telling you that certain products will prevent particular diseases, which is a fear-based approach, and they are more than happy to provide you with a litany. It is hardly arguable that what you refer to as your *healthcare system* is, in fact, focused on treating illness. So, it really ought to be called our *illness care system* since the care is focused on illness.

Most people – and dictionaries for that matter – seem to have the view that health simply means being free from illness or injury. But you know as well as I do that this is too simplistic. Health is much more than that.

Health is a state of complete mental, social and physical well-being, not merely the absence of disease or infirmity. ~ World Health Organization, 1948

But is that old World Health Organization (W.H.O.) definition that health professionals have been quoting since 1948 really what health means to you? They use the term "complete well-being" which suggests that you cannot be in a state of health unless everything is perfect, and it certainly includes, but is not limited to the notion of complete absence of any kind of illness. This is nonsense. And dangerous.

In 1986 the W.H.O. updated their definition when they created the Ottawa Charter for Health Promotion which suggested the following:

"Health is... a resource for everyday life, not the objective of living. Health is a positive concept emphasizing social and personal resources, as well as physical capacities."

So, *is* health a resource? In a sense it is. And..." *not the objective of living"*? This, too, is a very important concept for you when you consider what health means. If you reframe your thinking about health to see it as a personal resource, you can begin to focus on the kinds of health and life goals that aim to take you to points that are a means to living your life well to the end. After all, can you really say no to another resource? Despite the auspiciousness of the source of the notion that health is a resource (the W.H.O.), no one has paid much attention to this idea.

In 2007, a Canadian academic partnered with a human resources analyst for the federal government to publish a paper on how we can think about health as a resource. In that paper, they contend that "...health is a stock of biopsychosocial resources that people can draw on to participate in society." So, being healthy – whatever that means (and we'll get to that) – is what permits us to have a full life to the end.

Now, in the twenty-first century, we are constantly bombarded with messages suggesting to us a path to "wellness." Is this the same thing as health? Let's take a closer look at the wellness craze.

In 1979 storied American broadcaster Dan Rather introduced a special segment on his television news feature show on the latest health movement of the time by saying that the term wellness was a "word you don't hear every day." How times have changed!

With its roots in the 1950's, the modern wellness movement was, in fact, inspired by that 1948 definition of health as presented to the public by the World Health Organization. Anyone who studied medicine or nursing in the 1960's and 1970's was certainly inculcated to the work of an individual who happened to be an American biostatistician named Halbert L. Dunn (M.D., Ph.D.) who wrote a book called *High Level Wellness*. This book was required reading for many aspiring health professionals, especially nurses, back in those days. Dunn's ideas were, in some ways, revolutionary. He suggested that there are "Eight Points of High-Level Wellness." His eight points propose that to achieve this "high-level wellness" you have to be willing to do the following:

- Face inconsistencies in the way you think;

- Be open minded about others' points of view;

- Encourage others to express themselves freely;

- Adjust your personal views as necessary based on new input;

- Take your time with cultivating relationships that may be necessary to your life;

- Give credit to others when called for;

- Accept opportunities to serve others; and

- Offer freedom to those we love.

Not much of this sounds like the advice your current healthcare provider gives you, does it? However, if you look closely, you'll see a road map of sorts. Dunn focused on two elements: First knowing yourself, and second, maximising your potential *within the environment you find yourself*. This is important.

So, the concept of wellness in its purest, nascent form, was useful. However, the twenty-first century application of the term "wellness" has morphed into a worldwide industry worth somewhere in the vicinity of $4 trillion US dollars. Yes, *$4 trillion*. This includes industries such as beauty and anti-aging, nutrition and weight loss, fitness, and complementary medicine among others. Given that the beauty and anti-aging portion of this wellness boom is the largest, it suggests that you need to move beyond the concept of wellness to something perhaps more meaningful. But before we move toward embracing the real meaning of health in your life, we need to consider the newest media darling: self-care.

Throughout the 1980's and into the 1990's we were bombarded by pronouncements that we all needed "self-improvement." At that time, much of that self-improvement focused on achieving career success. Since the advent of so many digital devices in our lives, and the fact that we seem to be tuned into everyone else but ourselves for so much of our time, the movement toward twenty-first century self-improvement has turned to what the media influencers (see our discussion in Chapter 6) are now calling "self-care" which, as you might have figured out, is a fast-growing, quasi-health-related industry.

In a 2018 article in the *Harvard Business Review*, author Charlotte Lieberman suggests that our quest for self-improvement through self-care can border on obsession. For example, it seems that recent studies of Fitbit™ wearers indicate that the devices more often than not make the wearers feel guilty. She also suggests that the quest contributes to self-criticism. Her conclusion that "…there are infinite opportunities for personal growth, self-care, and genuine stress relief that don't require money or clenched fists…" suggests a more common sense approach to this forgotten land of health.

Forget the jargon. Forget all this self-care noise in your environment (remember to ask the question: who benefits most from this? You're likely to find that it is the marketer of the product or service, not you).

Rid yourself of the trendy gobbledygook: embrace the real meaning of health.

If life is the land of Oz, is health the Emerald City? I argue that it is not. Health is not the Emerald City, the destination; rather health is the Yellow Brick Road you take on your way to your final terminus. Like Dorothy, you need to decide what direction you'll take at each fork in the road, and know who your traveling partners really are or should be before the wizard makes the final reveal.

Do you really know what you want?

After more than four decades of practicing medicine, I've concluded that most people have no real idea of what they want out of their healthcare or – in many instances – their life. For example, have you really given any thought to what you want out of your health care beyond an immediate "fix"? Have you thought about how you would like to see your life's journey unfold, knowing that it is finite? I'm not talking about career aspirations or family goals or the meaning of life. I mean real, thoughtful, meaningful considerations of what your life will – and should – look like as you approach the end – whether that end is tomorrow or thirty years from now.

If you were to search online for help in figuring out these goals, what you'd find are reams and reams of web sites and life coach gurus who seem to think that what you're looking for is the purpose of your life. That's not what I'm talking about. Figuring out your purpose in life is a long-term project. If you're unable to come to a firm conclusion about this, it will likely frustrate you making you feel as if you have somehow failed. Consider this possibility: the purpose of your life is to have a life. Period. End of story. Feel better now? So, let's move on.

Rather than pondering the overwhelming questions, consider these ones:

- What do you want to see along the way toward your inevitable end?

- How would you like to feel along the way toward your inevitable end?

- Who would you like to have with you along the way to your inevitable end?

- Hypothetically, what would put a smile on your face as you lay dying?

The answers to these questions should take you some time to figure out. And when you have a few answers, you'll have a broad view of your life and health goals. Then you can figure out the specifics. Laugh, love, live, and if you're lucky, leave a legacy.

Just saying that you want to be healthy is useless to you, and to your doctor whom you might have the unfortunate desire to say this to. On the other hand, it is important to see your

Your goals are the road maps that guide you and show you what is possible for your life. ~ Les Brown

goals in a larger sense than those such as the following: I want to lose 30 pounds, or I want to run a marathon. These are not the kinds of road maps you need to navigate your highway to the end. You may very well accomplish those specific objectives, but they are not what will feed into the answers to the questions posed above.

Maybe you want to be resilient. That's a good road map. It suggests a number of activities, but it keeps things flexible. You aren't locked into training for a marathon, for instance. What happens if you break your leg? Can you not still pursue the overall goal of being resilient? Of course, you can, but you probably won't be running a marathon in the next few months.

Maybe you want to be comfortable. Maybe you would like to work longer, play longer, travel more? These are the kinds of things that might bring that smile to your lips as you lay dying. Think about it.

It's important to see your health as part of your big picture without succumbing to that existential torment that comes from trying to figure out your "purpose in life." The truth is that you cannot figure out whether or not you have achieved this type of true purpose until seconds before you die. At that point you can't do any more. If you get yourself so bogged down in trying to sort out your reason for existence, you'll miss the journey. You will find that, at the end, all along you already had what you were seeking. Remember Dorothy and her traveling companions?

Even big-picture goals are more like guideposts on your journey than they are destinations. Let's look at how you might find some authentic, doable goals.

COMMON SENSE GOALS: FINDING AND MAINTAINING BALANCE

My wife, who is a woman of a "certain age," as she likes to say, has always maintained specific life goals that are important to her. One of these goals that she uses along her own journey through life is *to maintain a youthful perspective on life*. This is an admirable goal in general for anyone who recognizes, and rightly so, that our bodies, and minds change as we move through life, but our perspective doesn't have to. It might even be a goal that resonates with you. Feel free to jot it down. In any case, this particular goal manifests itself in a variety of choices that my wife makes from her diet to her yoga to her love of learning new things, and even to her work to keep up to date with technology. However, occasionally, she falls out of *balance*.

Recently, she began to examine her skin in her magnifying mirror just a bit more often than usual, coming to the unfortunate conclusion that it seemed to be more lined, less clear and saggier than she remembered. This revelation spurred her to take stock of her skin care and cosmetic products, do some research and begin trying a variety of new products. Just as one product seemed to be working – it created another issue that required another product, and on and on until this otherwise sensible woman who prefers a more minimally stocked cosmetic drawer suddenly owned what looked a lot like a retail cosmetic counter full of partially used products. Then she developed an inflammation in one of her eyes that her ophthalmologist could find no cause for. That's when she had her Eureka! moment. Perhaps she was doing too much with her skin and needed to do less. That's when it occurred to her that she may have gone off the deep end with products putting her skin out of *balance*. But she was only able to deduce this because she understands one very important rule of maintaining balance: to find the centre of the fulcrum, you have to recognize that there is another diametrically opposite perspective from the one where you find yourself.

Remember this illustration from Chapter One?

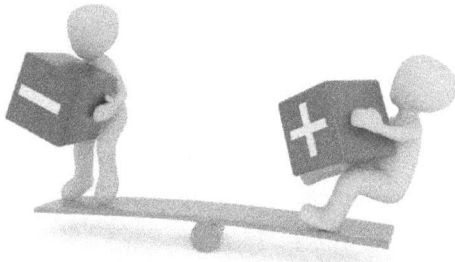

When I began the discussion of what it really means to find a common sense approach to life and health, I said that *balance* is the mechanism by which you apply your own common sense. If you overdo one thing, you have to balance that with more of the opposite, or less of the same. In my wife's case, she decided to go cold turkey and minimize her skin care to elements that have been recommended by her dermatologist (who has written a book on the subject of skin care) and stop using makeup entirely for a period of time to let her skin calm down. And this decision was made by a woman who would never leave the house without her foundation etc. But it was the only way she could begin to add in the essentials and get her regimen back in balance. She is still able to maintain her youthful perspective without succumbing to the bombardment from cosmetic companies that tell her that she needs a wide variety of products. She doesn't.

When you are figuring out the over-arching goals that will assist you in being most comfortable on your way toward the end of your life, it's important to consider that there are three important elements that have to be balanced for this to work.

- Your physical self,

- Your emotional self, and

- Your social self.

If you focus too much on physical goals while ignoring your emotional self, you will not be in balance. Just as you can't focus entirely on your social circumstances without considering your physical self. These pieces of who you are need to be in balance. Each of them overlaps, and a balanced *you* sits right in the middle where they all overlap.

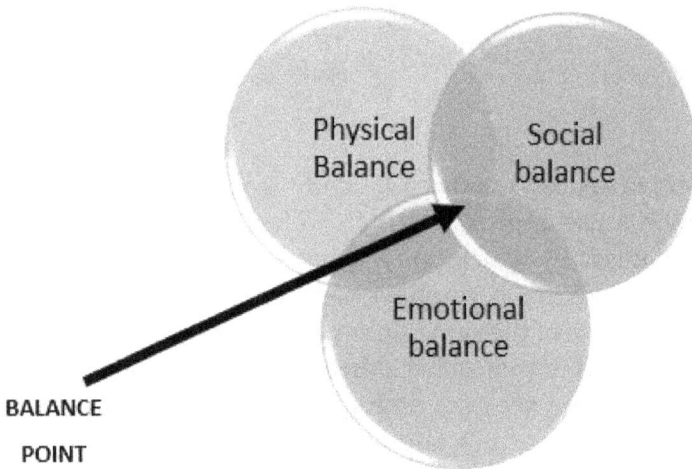

Physical Balance

Social balance

Emotional balance

BALANCE POINT

Remember that any goal you set must be flexible. If you are unable to adapt to changing circumstances, you'll have great difficulty in finding those balanced goals for your life – and rebalancing when you need to. My three grown children will be the first to tell you that one of my favourite quotes is by the Greek philosopher Heraclitus who is reputed to have said, "Nothing endures but change." It is something of a mantra in my life, and is a perspective I have shared with many patients over the years. Nothing stays the same, so if you fail to be flexible and adapt to those changing circumstances, you will not achieve the success you want along your journey. It's worth considering that nothing takes more of your energy than trying to keep things the same. Everything changes.

If you consider yourself to be fairly rigid, maintaining an inflexible approach to your life over time, I guarantee you that you will find yourself

> *No man ever steps in the same river twice, for it's not the same river and he's not the same man.* ~ Heraclitus

out of balance on numerous occasions. It is the tree that does not bend that gets uprooted in the storm.

Whether you like it or not, there will be many times in life that you have to change the path you are on as a result of insurmountable obstacles. Doing the same thing over and over and yet expecting different results is what has often been described as the definition of "insanity." (This quote has been variously attributed to Sigmund Freud, Albert Einstein and Mark Twain). Or as the *Urban Dictionary* puts it, "…doing the exact same fucking thing over and over again, expecting shit to change. That. Is. Crazy."

When you encounter those inevitable obstacles on your life's journey, whether they are specifically related to your health or your life in general, this could be your higher self giving you a nudge to change. That gentle – or occasionally not-so-gentle – nudge is an insight into how you should proceed. But this only works if you are prepared to listen then to adapt your personal life and health goals to deal with the obstacle. As you age, those health-related obstacles often present themselves more frequently – it is simply one of the vagaries of aging. You could refuse to see them and continue your life in exactly the same way you have conducted it in the past, but you do so at your peril. Consider maintaining some flexibility in your health goals. For example, if you run marathons in your forties, as you age you will likely notice that you have more injuries, aches and pains. If you continue to force yourself to run marathons in spite of these hints to stop, you will be less happy with your health than if you respected your body, and changed your activities.

Before I move on to helping you to figure out the resources you'll need to help you along the way, I'll finish this discussion of your goals by reminding you that the key to balance is moderation. Taking the extreme position when examining your own health maintenance and treatment activities is generally not the best approach. Remember the teeter-totter analogy. If you put a lot of weight and/or effort onto one side, something has to change on the opposite side to balance that weight or effort out. Consider what Greek philosopher Epictetus once said: "If one oversteps the bounds of moderation, the greatest pleasures cease to please."

> *The best and safest thing is to keep a balance in your life, acknowledge the great powers around us and in us. If you can do that, and live that way, you are really a wise man.* ~ Euripides

How to Figure Out the Resources You'll Need to Help You

One of the things that you probably already know for sure about life in general, and your health and health care in particular, is that you need resources to assist you along your path toward the end, regardless of where you currently stand on that journey. No one goes it alone forever. There are people in your life who are there to help, and there are people whose intervention – or interference, if you like – will only hinder your movement toward achieving your goals.

ADD PEOPLE WHO ARE...	SUBTRACT PEOPLE WHO ARE...
•helpful	•toxic
•knowledgeable	•negative
•caring	•narcissistic
•supportive	•obstructive

Here is a list of the kinds of people who will not be helpful to you and that you should ditch:

- People who don't understand your goals for your health and life;

- People whose interests are more about having you do what they do than what's right for you;

- People who don't listen to you;

- People who lie to you;

- People who support a victim mentality – whether in themselves or in you;

- People who demonstrate narcissism.

Here is a list of the kinds of people who will be beneficial to you in setting and achieving your goals:

- People with the genuine knowledge and skills you'll need to move along your path;

- People who listen;

- People who are genuinely interested in you and what's best for you;

- People who will tell you the truth even if it is not in their own best interest.

Apart from the people who will be helpful to you, you also need to figure out a way to access the resources you'll need along the way because, as I said, you can't always go it alone. Some of the resources you'll need might be the following:

- The healthcare system;

- Educational materials;

- Formal support systems.

One of the best paths to finding the appropriate resources will be the people you have in your life. They are resources in themselves. One of the most important of these resources will be your primary healthcare provider, a family physician for most of you. If you have the right family doctor, you'll be able to access many of the other helpful people and things that will support you on your way to achieving your goals.

In Chapter 10 I'll discuss how you can put common sense into action in your relationships with your healthcare providers – including your family doctor.

THE TWO MOST IMPORTANT WORDS IN THE ENGLISH LANGUAGE

Do you know what those two words are? I often joke with my wife that the two most important words in the English language for men are, "Yes, dear." And for children, "Yes, Mom." However, there are two others that over-ride even these important word duos: "I am…"

You'll recall that we had a fairly in-depth discussion in Chapter 5 about the power of your vocabulary, especially when referring to yourself. How you describe yourself can have compelling consequences for your life. So, whenever you begin a sentence with the two words "I am", you are about to put a label on yourself and that label can either help you or hinder you.

Consider the following possibilities:

- I am happy.
- I am healthy.
- I am strong.
- I am youthful.

…versus…

- I am unhappy.
- I am okay.

146

- I am weak.

- I am old.

Each of these words that follow "I am" – the label – tells a story about you – to you as well as to others. But there are other words that seem to have fewer polarizing possibilities, and yet how you interpret them and act on them can have consequences for your life.

Consider the following labels:

- I am overweight.

- I am fat.

- I am big.

- I am heavy.

Each of these labels carries with it a lot of baggage. Oprah (and others) would have you believe that you should always tell yourself that you're beautiful, ignoring the fact, obvious to you when you get on the scales, that you are also overweight, for example. Considering yourself to be beautiful at any weight may be a good thing for your mental health – and I support that – but if you do not also say "I am overweight", being honest with yourself, then you will never take any action to do something about being overweight which is both a health and life issue. Sometimes the relabeling can simply mean that you are ignoring a reality that you might be able to do something about if you used that label positively. It is worth considering.

Setting goals for your health and your life constitutes a good exercise in figuring out how you want to travel on your journey toward the end of your life. Being honest with yourself is the first step.

It might be wise to consider the words of tennis great Arthur Ashe who once said, "Success is a journey, not a destination. The doing is often more important than the outcome."

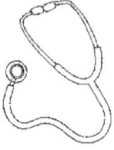

KEYS TO YOUR HEALTH GOALS

☑ Remember that health is one of your most important resources for assuring a good trip through life.

☑ Forget trying to figure out your reason for existence if you are interested in having a good life trip. (The truth is that you might just be living to be a proverbial spear-carrier in someone else's play, and that's okay if you enjoy the journey.)

☑ Focus on figuring out what you'd like that journey to be like and take steps to move in that direction.

☑ Find the balance point of moderation in your movement toward your goals.

☑ Be aware that you may not have all the resources you need to help you along the way; spend some time finding them.

☑ Be aware that some of the resources you currently have in your life may not be serving you well; rid yourself of them.

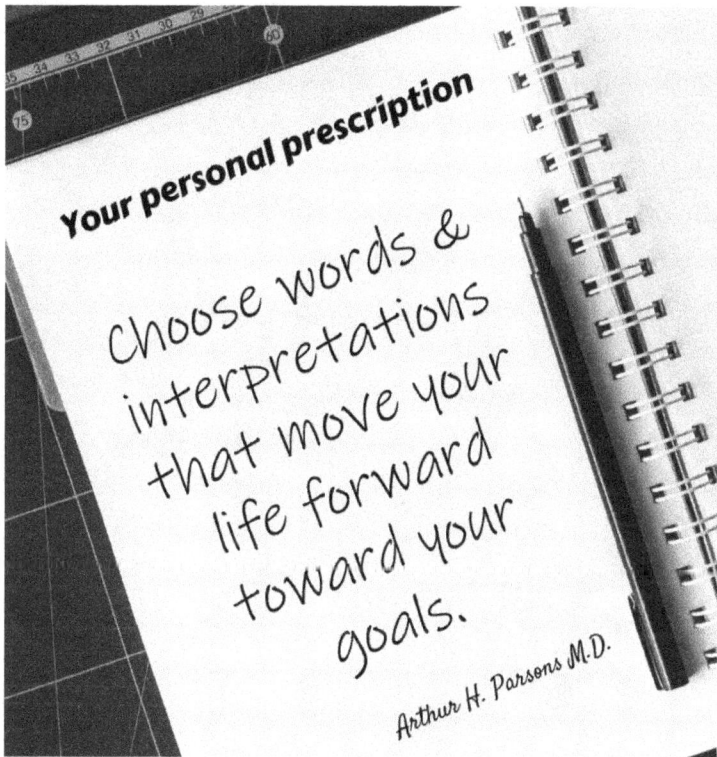

Your personal prescription

Choose words & interpretations that move your life forward toward your goals.

Arthur H. Parsons M.D.

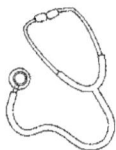

MEANWHILE BACK IN THE OFFICE

"KNOCK, KNOCK," PETE SAID rapping on Sherilynn's office door.

Dr. Sherilynn Fontaine was only a few years older than Pete, but had been a family physician for ten years. She had gone directly to medical school after her science degree, while Pete had spent two years on a Masters degree in microbiology then a further three years working in a lab before he had gotten that life-changing letter: his admission to med school. So, Pete often took advantage of what he and his colleagues referred to as "corridor consultations" to run things by one another – kind of like getting their own second opinions. He suspected that he did it more frequently than either Sherilynn or Tony, for sure, although even Tony still did it from time to time even after all his years in medicine. *Probably a good practice*, Pete thought.

"Have a moment for a consult?" he said as she looked away from her computer screen to see him standing in the doorway.

"Sure. What's up?"

Pete sat down on the examining table in her office and put the sheaf of papers that he had been holding down on the table's paper cover beside him.

"Do you have many patients who don't seem to trust their diagnoses?"

Sherilynn sat back in her chair and started to laugh. "Oh, Pete," she said, "that comes with the territory these days. Sometime I have days when I wonder if *anyone* actually believes their diagnoses any more. Especially when it doesn't match what they seem to want it to be."

"That's just it," Pete said, "I send someone out to a specialist, and when the patient has seen the consultant and the report comes back, if it doesn't match what they were expecting, they want another opinion, even if that opinion is not really an opinion, if you know what I mean. There is no doubt about it based on the tests that were done. That's fact, not opinion."

"Anything specific today?"

"Yeah. I have a patient in my office as we speak who's waiting for me to come back in to tell her that she can go to another rheumatologist about her supposed osteoporosis. The first one I sent her to – you know Sabina Patel, the best rheumatologist in the city – told her she doesn't need any medication at this point. The test results are unequivocal, and she doesn't need to see anyone else. I actually think it would be negligent of me to send her to someone else who will just tell her the same thing."

"Who's she been listening to?"

"I had hoped that it might be her medical team, but I guess I'm still a bit naïve about this stuff. Probably some television show or her friends."

"It's tough sometimes," Sherilynn said. "I think that's probably one of the most difficult aspects of medicine that I had to get used to when I started practice. No one prepares you for it. Sometimes when patients ask for tests that they don't need, for example, I find myself weighing the cost to the system versus the patient's psychological need for the test. I had three different people over the past two weeks ask me to send them for Vitamin D levels."

"Well, they're useless," Pete said. "They should be outlawed in my view."

"Of course, you know that, and I know that, but the patients seem to think that whoever is promoting it in the media knows more about it than we do. What I do know is that patients who continually want tests of dubious usefulness are less likely to accept our medical expertise about anything. All they need us for is to gain access to the system, and that's what they'll use us for. They're just not prepared to listen."

"So, I just have to get used to that?"

"Unless you want to take them on publicly. It's difficult. So, what are you going to do about the patient who's waiting in your office?"

"I think I'll send her to Kevin first. Maybe he can give her something to focus on rather than her desire for another opinion or those meds."

Kevin was the consultant dietitian who spent two days a week in their clinic seeing patients referred for dietary assessment and intervention.

"Good plan. Glad I could help!" Sherilynn laughed as Pete picked up his sheaf of papers and headed back to his own office.

~

Later that afternoon, after Pete had long dispatched his patient to the dietitian, he walked through the reception area from the file room when he caught a glimpse of a carefully wrapped, bright red scarf partially obscuring the face of the wearer. *That looks very elegant*, he thought as he passed. A few minutes later the red scarf was sitting in his examining room.

"Mrs. MacDonald, how nice to see you," he said sitting down. "What a lovely scarf that is."

Seventy-eight-year-old Judith MacDonald beamed. Her eyes were still bright and her smile contagious, although Pete knew that it masked a continuing struggle with a devastating diagnosis.

Judith had cancer, and things were not looking good at this stage. In fact, her latest report from her oncologist indicated that there were few options left, although they were willing to try some.

Together they reviewed her recent chemotherapy treatment which she told Pete would be her last. This was the reason she had come back to him, she told him, rather than going to her oncologist again. She wasn't going to need oncology services any longer.

"I know that my journey is almost over," she said, then brightened up. "But I'm not dead yet!"

Pete felt as if he had been struck in the chest. He had truly come to enjoy Judith's visits. Despite her cancer, she had been a ray of sunshine on the days she had come in to see him. While most of his cancer patients talked of waging a battle with their disease, of winning the war, of surviving the struggle, of fighting, fighting and more fighting, Judith had always taken a different – and in Pete's view – surprisingly refreshing view of this destructive disease. From the very beginning, Judith had characterized her illness as merely another chapter – albeit a difficult one – along her journey of life. When she had received the diagnosis, she was naturally distraught, but that feeling had quickly been replaced by her usual approach to life: stare at the situation in the face and figure out how to deal with it, because, as she had told her young family doctor on more than one occasion, "The glass is half full, after all, Dr. K. I need to focus on what's in it, not what's not there any more." And so, she had.

Judith had carefully researched her cancer, its treatment and prognosis then embarked on being the best patient possible when confronted with more and different treatment options. She had taken a brief foray or two into alternative approaches, always maintaining a healthy scepticism. This all happened over a ten-month period.

And all of this together had worked – until it didn't. And she knew it.

"I'm starting to get a bit annoyed by my daughter and her continual conversations – well, monologues really – about how she expects me to keep fighting, to win the battle then the war. To take no prisoners. What does she think this is? World War Three? Dr. K.," Judith clasped her hands in her lap and turned to look directly at Pete who hadn't yet found the right response to Judith's news. "Dr. K., when I first met you eight months ago, I thought – here's a newbie doctor who'll probably want to fight this battle with all the ammunition possible until I'm nothing but a shell of who I once was. But I've found you to be one of the only people in my clutch of resources who actually listens to me. I don't think they can teach that in medical school. I think it's part of who you are. Am I right?"

"Well, Mrs. MacDonald…"

Judith leaned over placing her frail hand on his arm. "I think you can start calling me Judith…Pete."

Pete was disarmed, as usual. He blinked at her. "Judith…I've always respected you and how in tune you always seem to be with yourself. I've actually been a bit daunted by how you seem to be able to accept –"

She stopped him. "No, Pete, I don't *accept* anything at first glance. I examine it to see where it will take me. I look at the alternatives and the approaches to getting to each of them, weighing whether or not I'm prepared to do what it takes. But I do this without rose-coloured glasses. I see more clearly than my daughter ever will. I know I'm dying, but she can't seem to get there with me."

"It's often hard, maybe harder, for those we leave behind."

Judith sighed. "I know. But her attitude is beginning to interfere with my life. Just last week we went out to dinner. I ordered a martini – you know those dirty ones with all the olives I love so much – anyway, her eyebrows shot up. She said something to the effect that alcohol was probably ill-advised in my condition. *Ill-advised*? In my *condition*? I should think being able to do whatever the f**k I want to at this stage would be very advised."

Pete blushed slightly, not expecting to hear such language from the elegant Mrs. Judith MacDonald. "Well, Judith," he said clearing his throat, "I think that you are the best judge of what's right for you at this point in your life's journey."

"Damn right!" she said, smiling. "Can you write that on a prescription pad so I can wave it in my daughter's face?"

CHAPTER EIGHT

COMMON SENSE IN ACTION: LEARNING TO USE YOUR INTELLECT AND INTUITION

"The three great essentials to achieve anything worthwhile are first, hard work; second, stick-to-itiveness; third, common sense."
~ Thomas Edison

WE HAVE NOW ESTABLISHED that if life were the Land of Oz, then health would not be the Emerald City, rather it would be the Yellow Brick Road. You are on that road whether you want to be or not, but where it takes you and how you travel are largely under your control. One of the controllable aspects of this journey is your selection of vehicles.

> *Everybody gets so much information all day long that they lose their common sense.* ~ Gertrude Stein

At their most fundamental, these vehicles fit into one of three categories: the health (read medical) care system, alternative (complementary/non-mainstream) medicine, and self-help, all of which I'll discuss in greater detail a bit later. The truth is that these days, you might want to consider a combination of all of the above. And, if these are the vehicles, then you need fuel to make them work.

Even those who choose to walk along their journey will need to fuel their bodies. The fuel you'll need is intellect and intuition which together add up to *common sense*. The purpose of this chapter is to provide you with a general framework for using common sense to figure out if any given approach – regardless of who suggests it to you – is worth including in your healthy life's journey. But first, you need to understand precisely what is meant by your personal *intellect*, then your *intuition*, and how they work together.

THIS THING CALLED INTELLECT

We all possess it, yet few of us have ever taken the time to consider what it is. And most importantly we fail to figure out how to leverage it for best personal results. Of course, I refer to the concept of *intellect*.

Searching for definitions of the term suggests that it has a number of characteristics:

- Intellect is a faculty of your mind.
- It is what guides your rational thought processes.
- It involves your ability to reason.
- It takes an objective rather than subjective approach to decisions.
- It helps you to figure out the objective "truth" about things.
- It is what permits you to come to the correct decision based on fact.

As you can see from the above list, applying your intellect to decisions you make about your health or anything else for that matter, may move you toward some kind of objective "truth" and this is something you need to learn to do, but it isn't the whole thing as you'll see. You need more.

Back in 1952, philosopher Wilmon Sheldon published an article in the journal *Philosophy East and West* on the topic of intellect, specifically on the differences between how the disciplines of science and philosophy view it. In his opinion, intellect is our instrument for "grasping reality." So, I submit to you that the first step in your decision-making process is being able to leverage your intellect to view the facts dispassionately, and to see unvarnished reality. This is important if you are eventually to apply your intuition appropriately.

> *To expect the unexpected shows a thoroughly modern intellect.* ~ Oscar Wilde

Leveraging your intellect begins with understanding what it is – its components. *Core intelligence* is another way that your intellect has been described. However, this is only helpful if you understand what makes up this core of intelligence in *you* specifically.

THE THEORY OF MULTIPLE INTELLIGENCES

American developmental psychologist and Harvard professor Howard Gardner has described our intellect in terms of *multiple intelligences*, which is a helpful way to consider your own intellectual strengths and weaknesses, and how you might capitalize on them. He has described eight types of intelligence that we all possess.

I.   Linguistic intelligence: Your ability to read, write and speak. For example, if this is your strength, you are probably good at crossword puzzles.

II. Logical-mathematical intelligence: Your ability to figure out patterns and numbers. If this is your strength, you are probably good at strategy games.

III. Bodily-kinaesthetic intelligence: Your ability to learn and process movement information. If this is your strength, you are probably a good dancer, able to learn choreography, or you are good at crafting or sewing.

IV.   Spatial intelligence: Your ability to remember images and the degree with which you remember your surroundings. If this is your strength, you can visualize the world in 3D and might be a good architect or engineer.

V.   Musical intelligence: Your ability to understand rhythms, sounds and patterns of sound. If this is your strength, you probably remember songs well and might play an instrument (or be a dancer).

VI.   Interpersonal intelligence: Your ability to understand and relate to other people. If this is your strength, you are good at verbal and nonverbal communication and understand others' emotions and motivations. If this is your strength, you may be good a resolving conflict and creating positive relationships.

VII.   Intrapersonal intelligence: Your ability to be reflective and understand yourself. If this is your strength, you have very well-developed self-awareness and might excel as a writer.

VIII.   Naturalistic intelligence: Your ability to see patterns in nature and are in tune with your environment. If this is your strength, you may be good at categorizing information and enjoy gardening or other nature pursuits.

It's probably clear to you as you read through the descriptions of these "intelligences" that we all possess all of them to some degree. Some are more developed in each of us than are others. If you're going to apply your intellect – your intelligences – to making good choices throughout the remainder of your life, a good first step would be to analyze yourself to determine your personal strengths and weaknesses. You can then capitalize on your strengths and take action to improve upon your weaknesses. The first step is self-awareness.

If you perceive that you have one well-developed, easy to access type of intelligence, be careful. You might find that you tend to interpret everything within the frame of this particular intelligence. For example, if you perceive that your logical-mathematical intelligence is superior to other intelligences – perhaps the only one you identify with – you will take that logical approach to everything regardless of other aspects of a situation that might be useful to you. The result of this kind of approach is that you will end up with a very unbalanced point of view.

In addition to the notion of multiple intelligences as described above, there are two more aspects of your personal intellect that you need to become familiar with and figure out how to mobilize before you can truly apply your common sense. These are:

- Analytical thinking, and

- Experiential intelligence.

IMPROVING YOUR ANALYTICAL THINKING

Analytical thinking is simply your ability to break down complex issues or problems into their more manageable pieces. For example, if you are faced with a major health problem, it is easy to be overwhelmed by the situation. Not being able to see it as anything but a huge, problematic whole will seriously hamper your ability to move forward – you will not be able to use common sense at all to move through it. If, however, you are able to analyze the situation carefully, breaking it down into its component parts (treatment options, care for your children, work problems that will inevitably arise, personal care etc.), then deal with each one individually, you will begin to make progress.

Some people are very good at this – it is one of their intellectual strengths. However, if it's one of your weaknesses, you can improve your analytical skills.

When was the last time you decided to learn something new? And this doesn't mean a major project like learning to play a musical instrument or returning to school to change careers. It could be small, like learning how to cook green beans perfectly. In fact, if you do take on a larger learning project, what you really need to focus on is learning one new thing at a time – and that improves your critical thinking skills. If you decide you'd like to learn repair the grout in your shower, you might begin by researching the kinds of grout available and learning their individual characteristics. Then you move on to watching a YouTube video about the process and buying the supplies you need. One step at a time. If you focus on learning one new thing every day, or even every week, this may help you to improve those critical thinking skills.

Most psychologists (and human resources coaches as it turns out) recommend various ways to do this. Here are a few suggestions of where to begin:

- *Read more*. If you're not in the habit of reading every day, now might be the time to start. Reading makes you think. If you need some external encouragement, join a book club. It doesn't matter whether you read fiction or nonfiction, just read about things you know little about.

- *Figure out how things work*. These days, this is as easy as going online and searching for videos that demonstrate everything from fixing your running toilet to baking a cake.

- *Keep a journal*. This is the place for you to write your thoughts about the situations you face. As you re-read these entries, you will begin to think about what they mean to you and how to deal with them piece by piece. My further advice: keep your journal to yourself. Don't blog about it for everyone to see and comment on. Don't post excerpts on Facebook. This is one time when social media is not your friend.

- *Take a course* either online or at your local university or library. This is an extension of learning something new every day, but on a larger scale. If this is the route you choose, be sure to focus on one lecture or section of the course at a time.

- *Commit to spending less time on social media.* Don't waste so much time living the lives of your friends. Live your own life in the real world.

What's interesting about improving your critical thinking skills is that this will help you not only on your life's journey, but also in other aspects of your life such as your career and in your relationships. It's worth spending some time on.

USING YOUR EXPERIENCE

For a long time, intelligence was considered to be inherent – in other words, it came strictly from within the individual. That meant that it was fixed at birth and you couldn't change it. However, we now know that there is more to your intellect than your genetic makeup. One very important way we develop our intelligence is through experience – and my view is that how and what we learn through experience becomes a part of our intellectual abilities.

In Chapter Two I discussed how you develop your attitudes and beliefs through a variety of "ways of knowing." I suggested to you at the time that one of the most powerful ways that we come to *know* things in our lives is via direct experience – empiricism. Although a young mother might tell

> *Intelligence is the ability to adapt to change.* ~ Stephen Hawking

a child that he should not put his hand on the stove top lest he get a burn, the child will have that notion forever etched in his psyche if he actually ignores Mom and tries it out – if he has the experience. The consequent burn will become a part of his experiential learning, and thus part of the intellectual material he can use for making decisions as he gets older. It is the same for you.

The problem these days in the era of the so-called "helicopter parent" is that the new generation of future adults may not be permitted to have some of the experiences from which they might learn these life lessons. Over-protection robs children and adolescents of some experiential learning that would prove useful in their adult decision-making.

You have experiences that you may, however, have failed to learn from, having not changed your behaviour in any way as a result. These experiences, then, do not become part of your intellect. However, if you have *changed your behaviour* in some way as a result of experiences, then you have truly learned something, and this real knowing is part of the intellectual capital you can use in future situations. In fact, one of the traditional definitions of "learning" is a change in behaviour. This is easily illustrated by looking at a typical classroom situation. Just because the teacher "teaches" something does not equate with the students learning it. If there is no change in their knowledge level, attitude or behaviour, then the students cannot be described as having learned anything. So, behaviour change, or adaptation really, is key.

We should not pretend to understand the world only by the intellect. The judgement of the intellect is only part of the truth. ~ Carl Jung

American psychologist Robert Sternberg, who developed his own theory of human intelligence(s), has suggested that, "Intelligent behaviour involves adapting to your environment, changing your environment, or selecting a better environment." This is a very important concept for you on your journey through life, and clearly requires some intellectual ability to accomplish. It is how you deal intelligently with new situations – circumstances in which you have never found yourself before. If you can use past experiences to figure out how to deal with new ones, you have applied your experiential intelligence. And like the little child who now knows to avoid hot surfaces, you can adapt your behaviour for more positive outcomes.

One caveat: This cannot be applied equally to interpersonal relationships. For example, if you had a problem with what you view as a particular type of person, you may conclude that you will have an equivalent kind of experience with anyone else you perceive to be the same. This is what we call prejudice.

But do you really understand what it means to *adapt*? It simply means to change something to fit a new situation – a new set of circumstances. If you were to go blind in one eye, your remaining eye would eventually adapt to its new reality. That is, to some extent, built into the human physical condition. However, you might also have to adapt to new ways of doing things, and if you have difficulty with that aspect of losing the vision in one of your eyes, you will not be able to function optimally. Albert Einstein, who knew a thing or two about intelligence and intellect, is often quoted as having said, "The measure of intelligence is the ability to change." Who can argue with such an eminent thinker? If there is one lesson in this entire book for you it has to be this:

> The ability to adapt to life's changes is the surest way to smooth your journey.

However, you are more than your thought processes.

WHY CAN'T *YOU* BE THE FUNDAMENTAL VEHICLE THROUGH WHICH YOU CREATE HEALTH?

A "gut feeling" is a bit of a cliché, yet there is some truth to it. Trusting a feeling within yourself that tells you something is right for you or wrong for you is a powerful force that cannot be ignored (nor can it be used in

The world is a teacher to the wise man, and an enemy to the fool. ~ Ancient wisdom

isolation). This is part of what we refer to as *intuition*. Your intuition can be applied to situations you find *yourself* in, but you cannot apply your intuition to others – and don't even try. Learning when and how to use your intuition is an important step in your decision-making. Let's begin by figuring out what intuition is and how it manifests itself.

Whenever people talk about intuition, the word instinct always seems to play a part. But are they the same thing? Do you really have "instincts" like our animal friends do? And, if so, how can you ignore them? Business consultant Francis Cholle, author of *The Intuitive Compass: Why the Best Decisions Balance Reason and Instinct*, differentiates among the three concepts of gut feeling, instinct and intuition in the following way:

> *"...Instinct is our innate inclination toward a particular behaviour (as opposed to a learned response)... gut feeling – or a hunch – is a sensation that appears quickly in consciousness (noticeable enough to be acted on if one chooses to) without us being fully aware of the underlying reasons for its occurrence...Intuition is a process that gives us the ability to know something directly without analytic reasoning, bridging the gap between the conscious and nonconscious parts of our mind, and also between instinct and reason..."*

Notice that he suggests that intuition is a "process" that we use without *analytical reasoning*. After our discussion about intellect, critical thinking and rational reasoning above, you might have concluded that this is all you need for decision-making. But it isn't. You need both of these approaches.

Sometimes your intuition tells you something about what is going on in your body. You have no hard data to support this sense. You have not "Googled" various aspects of what you think is going on, you have not discussed it with anyone – you are just accessing that unconscious part of yourself that is telling you

The intuitive mind is a sacred gift and the rational mind is a faithful servant. We have created a society that honours the servant and has forgotten the gift. ~ Albert Einstein

to take action. You might consider listening. Be careful, though, that the true cause of your gut feeling is not anxiety or fear. True gut feelings, even if the results could be negative – a feeling about an impending disaster for instance – are not originally felt as fear. The fear comes after the inevitable analysis of that feeling.

One of the things that your intuition does is permit you to become more attuned to your physical and emotional states. If you look at emotions as flags that indicate that something needs attention, the tail does not end up wagging the dog, and these emotions do not control you. This may help you to find the best resources to support your journey. But it requires you to look and listen, and to do this, you often have to be quiet. Many people find meditation helps them to tap into their intuition. This is that quiet time when you may be able to pay attention to what's going on in your interior. If you don't like the idea of meditation, just sit still for a while and be quiet.

So, how do you apply your intuition? It's not that you have to make a choice: **reason + logic + evidence** versus **instinct + intuition + gut feeling**: they are all important. That's the common sense approach.

COMMON SENSE DECISION-MAKING

In a 2012 book called *Intuition in Medicine,* author Hillel Braude who is both a physician and a philosopher, suggests that intuition is a kind of common sense reasoning. My experience tells me that this is only partly true. Although I do believe that in healthcare in general, and medicine in particular, little credence has been given to the role intuition plays in healthcare decisions, I also believe that leaving all your decision-making up to gut instinct is foolish. Equally as unwise is taking the linear, rational, scientific approach on its own under most circumstances. Neither one alone can be called common sense. Whenever you apply your intuition to your decision-making without a dose of rationality, the decisions might be gut-based, but they are often incomplete. You need to get into the habit of mobilizing both your critical thinking abilities alongside your intuitive senses. Both are a part of your common sense.

TRAVERSING THAT FORGOTTEN LAND OF "HEALTH"

Now that we've established that your best approach to making decisions about your onward journey is to use your intellect/rational reasoning in conjunction with your intuition/instinct, the next step is to apply that to figuring out what vehicles will serve you best.

Intuition/
instinct

Intellect/
rational
reasoning

Common
sense
decisions

Let's examine the three broad categories of the vehicles you have available to you. As you consider each of them, remember that common sense tells you that you do not have to choose only one. In fact, doing so might be a reckless decision.

Science-based western medicine: This is the approach to your health and healthcare that you will receive from your average Western-trained doctor, nurse, nurse practitioner, even midwife. The approach is evidence-based and largely rational. You already know, however, based on our discussion in Chapter 6 of being careful about whom you listen to, that you do need to use some common sense even in the selection of experts to assist you along the way.

Alternative or complementary medicine (as we currently define it in the West): This is a more difficult category to define, although in the West, we do tend to lump everything that isn't "science-based Western medicine" into this group. In 2014, Dr. Mel Borins, a family physician and faculty member at the University of Toronto, published a book titled *A Doctor's Guide to Alternative Medicine: What Works, What Doesn't, and Why*. The book suggests that "alternative medicine" isn't really alternative at all these days, but that it has been called alternative because it has not been included in classical, Western medical education. Further, and this is important to help you understand why your family physician might be less than enamoured of your decision to take a fist full of homeopathic "medicines" instead of the medication he or she is recommending, Dr. Borins suggests that "...doctors worry that their patients may get into difficulty when taking an unregulated drug [or therapy] or they may delay receiving medical treatment that could improve their health or even be life-saving."

Remember, if you are choosing an alternative or complementary approach to your health care, you might not be able to rely on traditional, Western medicine to help you if you get into difficulty since so little may be known about it. Buyer beware. And, as he mentions, and we discussed in Chapters Three and Four, there is potentially a 30% placebo effect in any case whenever you believe in a drug or treatment's efficacy. What modalities fall into this category?

Alternative or complementary approaches cover a lot of territory. Some of them are sounder than others, however, their reliability, efficacy and safety are outside the purview of this discussion. The following are a few of the increasingly large number of alternative approaches you might consider:

- Traditional Chinese Medicine
- Osteopathy
- Chiropody
- Naturopathy

- Homeopathy
- Ayurveda
- Herbalism

If you refer to our discussions on being careful who you listen to in Chapter Six, and our discussion of intuition and intellect earlier in this chapter, you may be able to apply common sense to any decisions you might make about using these vehicles.

Self-help: The Merriam-Webster dictionary defines self-help as "…the action or process of bettering oneself or overcoming one's problems without the aid of others…" and this especially refers to choosing to avoid the help of professionals. This often does not mean actually going it alone; rather it means finding out information for yourself, often from non-expert peers.

These non-experts are often those patient-advocacy groups that we considered in Chapter Six. Many people find solace – and information – from their peers who are others facing the same or similar diagnoses. Common sense should now tell you that even if you share a diagnosis with someone, you are an individual with a different physical and emotional make-up so your experience of the disease will be different. People have different, deeply personal, reasons for starting or joining patient self-help groups.

One of the most egregious problems with self-help groups, however, is that they serve to reinforce certain mentalities. Remember when we discussed the "victim" and "survivor" mentalities? These words are the very labels that you'll hear again and again in the self-help movement.

Years ago, my sister-in-law was diagnosed with breast cancer. It was a small tumor which she had removed followed by some radiation and five years of the drug Tamoxifen™. During that time, she attended some breast cancer support groups and even volunteered with breast cancer patients for a few years. Then she stopped all of that. When asked why, her response was, "Because it keeps me thinking about myself as a cancer 'victim.' I'm just a person who used to have breast cancer." Long-term association with these support groups didn't work for her, and there are many others like her who have difficulty getting themselves disentangled when this kind of self-help ceases to provide further benefit.

Other members may try to persuade you to stay. Be aware also that even if the self-help group is a virtual one, the pressure to stay might still be there. In general, beware of the self-help approach. There may be aspects of it that are useful to you for a period of time, but remember that it may become problematic for you.

My personal view of self-help is that reading and learning on your own about approaches to dealing with life then choosing ideas that resonate with you can help you to move forward on your journey. Not all self-help requires groups, though.

WHO WILL YOU CHOOSE TO ACCOMPANY YOU?

Once you have selected the vehicles that you will use on your journey, you need to consider the individuals who will accompany you. This follows directly from the vehicles: traditional, Western medicine offers you people who practice in that realm and so on. In Chapter 10 we'll consider the relationships you develop with these individuals, but right now, just consider the myriad options available to you. Here are some of them:

- **Physicians**
  - o Your family physician, various specialists
- **Other mainstream health-care providers**
  - o Nurse practitioners, midwives, pharmacists, dietitians, physiotherapists, occupational therapists
- **Friends, relatives**
  - o Immediate family, best friends, extended family, online "friends"
- **Online influencers**

Parsons

o Bloggers, tweeters, Instagrammers, YouTubers, Facebookers etc.

As you consider all of this, remember that *your intellect, intuition and your common sense are often overshadowed by your emotions when it comes to decision-making regarding your health and healthcare.* Many people are unable to let go of their decision to be miserable. Whether you elect to see it this way or not, I submit to you that being miserable is a choice. Spend some time thinking about this. This is a prime example of emotion over intellect, and it has consequences in your life.

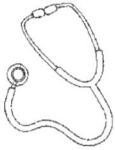

KEYS TO USING YOUR INTELLECT AND INTUITION

☑ It's important to evaluate your intellectual strengths and weaknesses.

☑ If your analytical thinking skills are lacking, take steps to improve them.

☑ Learn from your experiences.

☑ Listen to your intuitive nudges, then evaluate them.

☑ Use your intellect in concert with your intuition to make common sense decisions.

☑ Consider carefully what Western medicine has to offer you before dismissing it.

☑ Tread carefully when choosing alternative or complementary approaches.

☑ Don't let fear control your decision-making.

172

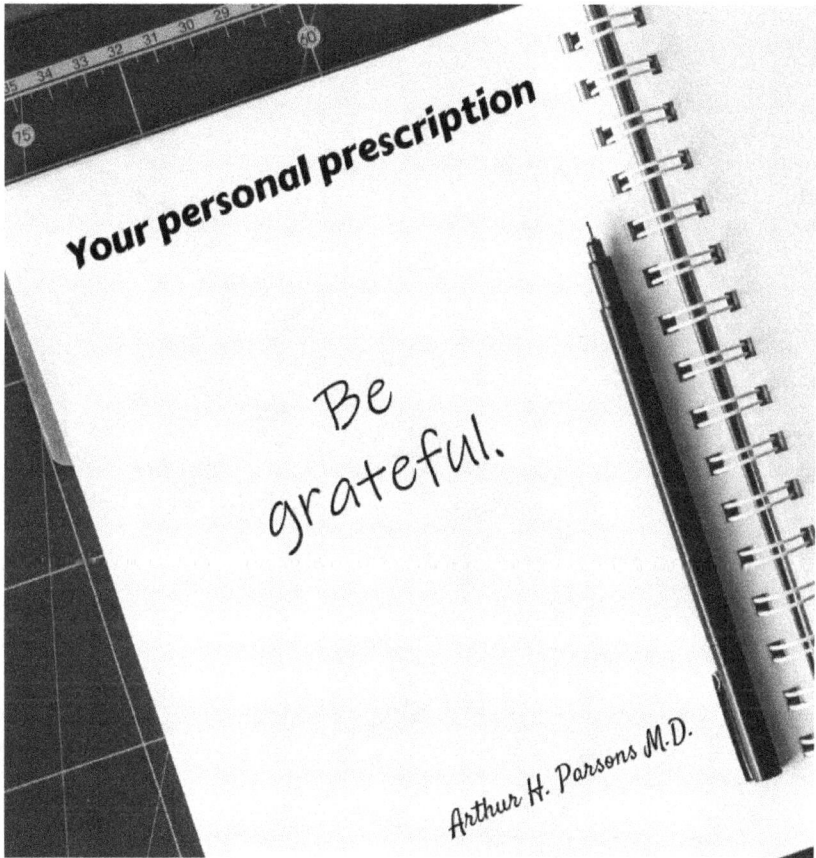

CHAPTER NINE

COMMON SENSE IN ACTION: DEALING WITH OBSTACLES AND SETBACKS

"You may not realize it when it happens, but a kick in the teeth may be the best thing in the world for you." ~ Walt Disney

THE BEST LAID PLANS, and all that. Stuff happens. We all get off course from time to time. When it comes to your health and your health care, there is little doubt that as we age, as our bodies age, things will change. And if you can adapt to those changes and deal head on with obstacles such as unexpected illness by using your common sense skills, you can improve your quality of life as you move along the journey toward that inevitable terminus.

There's an old adage that was popular back in the late twentieth century among self-help, life-improvement gurus. In fact, it was Henry Ford who actually said, "Obstacles are those frightful things you see when you take your eyes off your goals." Ford was clearly suggesting that you need to focus on your goal single-mindedly, or risk being frightened by obstacles, thus putting you off course. I am going to suggest to you that although it may work in business, this isn't an entirely helpful approach to take on your life journey. Being put off course might be the most important direction you could take at a certain point in that journey.

For centuries religious figures and philosophers alike have argued whether humans live a life that is pre-destined, or

175

whether life is a result of the choices we make. In addition, others believe that while some aspects of life are pre-destined, we have control over other parts by exercising free will. This latter approach is a true paradox that can be difficult to understand, but it is perhaps the best way to consider your path. Further, this approach allows you to see obstacles in your way differently.

If you, like many of my past patients, are having difficulty getting your head around this double-sided idea, perhaps the way I have always explained this to my patients (and my children, I might add), might help.

Life is like a large room. There is a door at one end through which you enter (birth), and a door at the other end through which you are designated to leave (death). Around the room there are other doors designated for others to leave through. Somewhere on that floor there is a path connecting your entrance and exit doors. Unfortunately, this path is covered over with multiple square tiles obscuring your way ahead. Although the path is there, somewhere underneath, you can't see it. But you can find it. You have a choice as to which tiles you remove, and in what order, to uncover that path. The problem that you may run into is that you remove tiles until you get sidetracked by someone else, and become involved in that person's path, forgetting your own journey and ending up exiting through their door, possibly prematurely. Or, you come up against a place on a wall that does not have an exit door. Despite this, and against all common sense, you keep pushing against or moving along that wall rather than back tracking, and improving the possibility that you will get back on track and find your right path. It is true that you can push along the walls or follow a path destined for someone else, and you may eventually find your exit, but it will not be a pleasant journey.

For anyone who skis, you might consider the analogy that life is like a mogul hill. Your predestined path is downhill, even if it is on a stretcher. The conditions depend on when you ski it. You have options. But each time you travel down the hill facing those moguls, there is really only one path that you take on that run. Thus, you are predestined, but you also have choice.

When you are on the right path things seem to be easy and you are "in flow" enjoying your journey. If you don't feel like yourself or you are not in flow, this is a message from you to you, so pay attention and make different choices. Remember, if you want to *change* some things in your life you have to *change* some things in your life!

When it comes to life's so-called obstacles, the common sense approach requires figuring out what the obstacle means in your life, and whether or not it really is a setback. It might well be an opportunity for change that you should not miss. Let's begin by figuring out what I mean by obstacles and the roles they can play in your life, keeping in mind that obstacles are not always obvious. Then I'll explain ways you might be able to turn obstacles into opportunities.

DEFINING AN "OBSTACLE"

There is little doubt that life's journey is rarely smooth: obstacles are an unavoidable part of life. No one is immune. The dictionary definition of an obstacle suggests that it is something that impedes, hinders or blocks progress. So, if an obstacle might *block* your path, it doesn't necessarily *have* to do so. It may only *impede* it or *hinder* your progress, or even slightly change your course.

Popular business blogger Ryan Holiday relates a version of an old Zen story that illustrates how an obstacle might be viewed in different ways. He tells the story of a

In the face of an obstacle which is impossible to overcome, stubbornness is stupid. ~ Simone de Beauvoir

king who grew concerned that his people had become too soft and entitled and he wanted to teach them a lesson:

> *"His plan was simple: He would place a large boulder in the middle of the main road, completely blocking entry into the city. He would then hide nearby and observe their reactions. How would they respond? Would they band together to remove it? Or*

177

would they get discouraged, quit, and return home? With growing disappointment, the king watched as subject after subject came to this impediment and turned away. Or, at best, tried half-heartedly before giving up. Many openly complained or cursed the king or fortune or bemoaned the inconvenience, but none managed to do anything about it. After several days, a lone peasant came along on his way into town. He did not turn away. Instead he strained and strained, trying to push it out of the way. Then an idea came to him: He scrambled into the nearby woods to find something he could use for leverage. Finally, he returned with a large branch he had crafted into a lever and deployed it to dislodge the massive rock from the road. Beneath the rock were a purse of gold coins and a note from the king, which said:

The obstacle in the path becomes the path. Never forget, within every obstacle is an opportunity to improve our condition."

One point of view suggests that always seeing obstacles as blocks is nonsense. Imagination and creativity might permit moving the obstacle, but I'm going to suggest to you that they are not all meant to be moved. Stay with me here.

Consider the following scenario that I have used countless times with hypnosis patients:

You are traveling along your path when you, like the travelers in the Zen story, come upon a boulder blocking your path. You examine the situation and eventually find a way around it. A little farther on, you happen upon a rock slide in your way. With great difficulty, you manage to crawl your way over it. Eventually you come to a small river, but the bridge has been destroyed. You wade in and swim across although it is a difficult swim in the rushing water. Finally, on the other side, you round a bend in the road and are faced with…the Grand Canyon. Then you realize: Wrong path! If you had been more attuned to yourself, you might have realized much earlier that this was not your path.

ROLES THAT OBSTACLES CAN PLAY IN YOUR LIFE

If obstacles – in both your path to good health and your life's journey – are unavoidable components of a life well lived, then it's important to figure out what roles they might play.

In general, obstacles on your health's path fall into two broad categories: obstacles presented by the expected and normal effects of aging, and those presented by unexpected illnesses of various causes, either acute or chronic, or accidents. Whether normal or not, whether expected or not, these obstacles are setbacks that can have a variety of meanings and play different roles. The two most important roles that they play are as signposts and as warnings.

Signposts: One of the most important roles that perceived obstacles play in your life is as signposts. Just as a signpost along a road provides you with information and direction, these obstacles also very often have such direction embedded in them if you are prepared to look and accept their direction. They can provide information on what is going to happen or what is supposed to happen in your life. If you are able to interpret their meaning, these signposts can help you to make good decisions about your health and your life. If you see a potential signpost as just another obstacle in your way, you will miss out on an important opportunity to improve your journey.

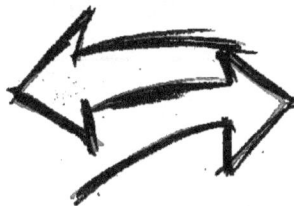

Warnings: Another important role that so-called obstacles can play in your life and health is as a warning. Unlike a signpost that provides general information and direction, a warning helps you to see potential danger. You may not yet have enough information to determine the direction you should take or the decisions you should make, but this warning ought to stop

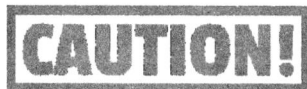

you from moving ahead in the same manner that you have been until you deal with that threat.

There is, of course, one further obstacle as some people see it. This is not an obstacle at all – it is the ultimate, full stop sign. It is the stop sign that everyone faces, cannot be overcome and must be accepted. It is death.

Remember:

- **Obstacles may not always have to be overcome.**
- **Obstacles may force you onto a different path (and that's okay).**

RECOGNIZING OBSTACLES: THEY'RE NOT ALWAYS OBVIOUS

At this point, it may occur to you that obstacles are always obvious: the cancer diagnosis, or the changes in your body as you age, for example. However, as much as these may pose challenges for you – and everyone else – some of the obstacles in your way, impeding your journey are not always quite so obvious. Here are some of the less obvious obstacles that may result in setbacks, or worse, if ignored or not recognized in the first place.

SITUATIONS OR CRISES IN YOUR FAMILY OR WORK LIFE: Negative situations in your everyday life or career, for example, can be major obstacles on your road to a good life. Common sense tells you that these cannot be ignored. If you remember our discussion of the relationship between mind and body in Chapter 4, it should be clear to you that how you think about these situations can have a major impact on your health.

PEOPLE: It should come as no surprise to you at this point in our discussion of common sense approaches to improving your health, that some of the people in your life might actually be obstacles to your good health. These days, most psychologists refer to these as *toxic people*, and they can be family members, acquaintances, so-called friends (either real or online), co-workers, bosses, and even children.

Dr. Abigail Brenner, writing in *Psychology Today*, identifies eight characteristics that may be signposts for you that you are dealing with someone who is toxic for you (remember, that someone who is toxic for you, may not be toxic for others). Here are some of the signs you need to be aware of as you consider whether or not certain people in your life are, indeed, obstacles that you have to deal with.

- Manipulative people;
- Judgmental people;
- People who refuse to take responsibility for their own feelings;
- People who never apologize, even when they clearly ought to;
- Inconsistent people;
- People who make you defensive;
- People who are uncaring, interested only in themselves.

There are also a few more clues that you are dealing with a toxic person. These people are not honest with you, they cannot forgive and forget and they always need to be right. If you have people in your life who are always surrounded by drama, take a step back: these individuals may be causing you more problems than you think. But what if a person you identify as toxic is someone whom you believe cannot be cut out of your life completely? For example, your toxic mother-in-law may be causing you problems, but as long as you are married to her offspring, she will always be a part of your life. You can, however, minimize contact and protect yourself by first being honest with yourself that she is toxic to you. You then need to figure out if she is a signpost or a warning and take appropriate action. When you take action, you regain some control.

THINGS IN YOUR OWN HEAD: Make no mistake, *you* might be the biggest obstacle on your own life and health journey. The two most important internal obstacles are *worry* and *fear*.

> *Worry never robs tomorrow of its sorrow, it only saps today of its joy.* ~ Leo Buscaglia

Worry is that feeling of anxiety that you have when thinking about things that are not actually real at the present moment. If you are simply thinking about the diagnosis that your doctor has just presented you with, you are probably ruminating and trying to process. However, the moment you begin to consider questions like, *How will I respond to the treatment? Or What will my family do if I get sicker?* You are now considering things that are not current problems. You are worrying, and worry can cause you more health problems than the original diagnosis.

One of the most problematic kinds of noxious worrying that my patients have exhibited is worrying about a diagnosis before it is made. For example, when a woman has breast biopsy because she's found a tiny lump in her breast, she will usually begin to worry that she has breast cancer, even before a diagnosis. Then, when the report comes back as benign, she has already made herself sick by worrying. Her common sense should suggest that she is no more likely to have cancer this week than she did last week before she found the lump. Perhaps reframing to consider that it might be benign would be better, but that doesn't align with the narrative women hear over and over in the media. Perhaps it's time to ignore the health media! If you are going to tell yourself a story, because this is what you are doing in these kinds of situations, commit to telling yourself one that is more advantageous to you.

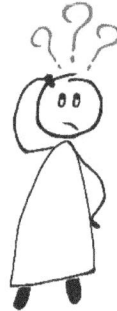

At this point you might be thinking that worry and fear are the same thing. They are not. Worry is a thought process focused on situations that are not yet real – and may never be. Fear, on the other hand, is that feeling you have about the realities of your life. This is an important distinction if you are to deal with these two related internal processes that can both be obstacles on your path. Remember that old adage: *worry is tomorrow's cloud pulled over today's sunshine*. It's worth considering the two general categories of things we worry about: those that you can do something about, and those that you cannot do anything about. Worrying about things you can't change is a complete waste of your time and energy. Worrying will certainly not change anything. Worrying about those things you can change is nonsensical: do something about them!

It is not the end of the physical body that should worry us. Rather, our concern must be to live while we're alive - to release our inner selves from the spiritual death that comes with living behind a facade designed to conform to external definitions of who and what we are. ~ Elisabeth Kubler-Ross

---

One of the most noxious aspects of fear is that it keeps you from taking action to make a difference. It often paralyzes you. A certain amount of fear is natural – and healthy. However, fearing something that is outside your control simply morphs into worry. On the other hand, if it is related to something within your control, then you can harness that fear and make changes.

It's not always easy to see that a perceived obstacle is in reality simply a road sign. It helps to gain some perspective by stepping away from proximity to the obstacle. In that way, you can see it with fresh eyes. Sometimes, it also helps to discuss the obstacle with a trusted healthcare provider (more about that in the next chapter).

HOW TO REFRAME, REFOCUS AND USE THE OBSTACLES: APPLYING COMMON SENSE

Here are some questions that you can ask yourself as you try to deal with potential obstacles in your path:

- Are there other routes to living well on the road to termination?

- Can I reframe how I see the obstacle?

- Is it possible for me to accept this and be happy about it?

- How can I be in the present moment, accept the present moment, and appreciate the present moment for what it is?

- Is it possible for me to express gratitude for what this obstacle might offer me? (Remember that gratitude is not for others' benefit, rather for your own benefit – that's what gratitude is all about.)

- Can I find a way to feel at peace?

- To whom can I express love?

- How can I find the joy in this situation?

You cannot control everything that happens to you in your life, nor can you control the obstacles in your path. However, you can reframe how you see them and refocus your attention. Reframing an obstacle as a sign, with a personal interpretation that is meaningful to you, allows you to move forward.

Perhaps it would be wise to remember the wisdom of spiritual leader Eckhart Tolle who said: *"Most people treat the present moment as if it were an obstacle that they need to overcome. Since the present moment is life itself, it is an insane way to live."*

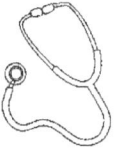

Keys to Dealing with Obstacles and Setbacks

☑ An obstacle in your path can become your path.

☑ Not all obstacles need to be removed.

☑ Obstacles can act as signposts or warnings.

☑ Not all obstacles are outside yourself.

☑ Take a step back from a perceived obstacle to figure out its real meaning.

☑ Worry and fear are two of the most problematic internal obstacles.

☑ You can reframe how you see an obstacle.

☑ Being in the present moment is probably the most important action you can take when faced with an obstacle.

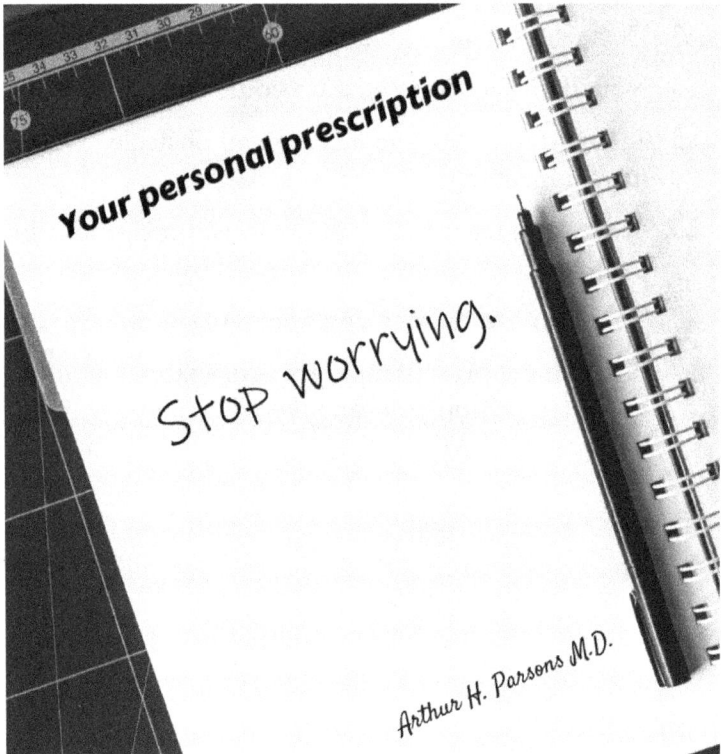

CHAPTER TEN

COMMON SENSE IN ACTION: RELATING TO YOUR DOCTOR AND OTHER HEALTHCARE PROVIDERS

"Some people think that doctors and nurses can put scrambled eggs back into the shell." ~ Dorothy Canfield Fisher

WOW! THERE IS SUCH AN EXTRAORDINARY AMOUNT of material written for health professionals on how to create a therapeutic relationship with a patient and how to communicate within that relationship! Guess what? There's very little on how a patient can communicate with care givers. But since your family physician or other primary healthcare provider is your access point into the healthcare system, it just makes sense that this relationship will be of prime importance.

If you've ever wondered what doctors learn in medical school about cultivating good patient relationships, you're not alone. But even as medical schools have become more concerned with teaching these so-called soft skills to budding physicians, it's equally as true that patients have given little thought to their own role in helping to cultivate great relationships with their healthcare providers. And if we are being completely honest, any kind of a relationship, if it is to work well, has to be two-sided. It's not all up to the patient – nor is it all up to the doctor. You cannot command complete control over the relationship since you're only one-half of it, but you certainly can make a difference by considering a common sense approach.

I'll begin by helping you to understand us – your healthcare professionals. Then we'll examine the elements of a good relationship with your healthcare providers and how common sense can guide the development of a great therapeutic relationship that will enhance your life's journey.

UNDERSTANDING HEALTHCARE PROFESSIONALS

Do you have faith in your healthcare providers? In your doctors? In a 2010 American study, 70% of respondents indicated that they trust their doctors, with the numbers slightly higher for respondents over age 65, and slightly lower for those under age 50. In early 2018, author Dhruv Khullar wrote a piece for in the *New York Times* titled: "Do You Trust the Medical Profession?" In it he indicated that although back in 1966 more than 75% of Americans said they had "great confidence" in their medical leaders, by 2018 that number had dwindled to 34%. A lack of confidence in the medical profession would come as no surprise to currently practising physicians. It is increasingly becoming the era of the second opinion – and that second opinion just as frequently comes from a non-expert such as a friend, relative or a post on Facebook, as it does from a real, qualified medical professional. It's hard for physicians not to perceive that their relationships with patients have eroded over the years.

The truth is that how physicians are perceived by members of the public has changed dramatically in the past 50 years. When I began medical school in the 1960's, the physician was regarded with a degree of respect based on his or her education and expertise. This was not a reverence; rather it was a distinct value placed on the expertise that the physician brought to the table – to the relationship. At least it permitted a sense of mutual respect that became the basis for the successful therapeutic relationship. By the time forty-five years of medical practice had come and gone, and I was winding down toward retirement, I often reflected on how things had changed. And not all for the better. That respect had somehow devolved into contempt, often a simmering-under-the-surface disdain. Whereas I welcomed the partnership of an involved patient

Sometimes, the best thing we can do for our patients is to tell them what the best behaviour is and then negotiate something they can live with. ~ Dr. Nancy Dickey

who does research and brings thoughtful questions into the discussion, I began to resent patients arriving at the door, pages printed off the internet in hand, demanding that I change my approach to conform with what the internet influencers were saying or merely what the patient wanted. If that made me defensive, I don't apologize. It was never a matter of wishing the patients would simply sit and accept everything that I said; rather it was a matter of expecting that at the very least my opinion, based on considerable knowledge and expertise (and knowing when I needed to consult further) would be valued by the patient.

When twentieth-century American medical education reformer Abraham Flexner said, "Medical education is not just a program for building knowledge and skills in its recipients... it is also an experience which creates attitudes and expectations," he was referring to one very important aspect of the education of any specific profession. We learn more than the hard, medical knowledge necessary to care for patients in our practices. We are also socialized into a profession. This is important for patients to understand since that professional socialization is still a part of medical education, but it has changed. Indeed, this is part of the education in any professional field.

The physicians graduating from medical school in the twenty-first century are different from those who graduated in the previous one. Relating to older physicians may be different than relating to younger ones. If you are older yourself, you will feel this most acutely because of your own years of experience with medical professionals.

These days doctors feel pressure from a number of areas. First, there is considerable pressure on your doctor from medical regulatory bodies. This is both a blessing and a curse for patients. As a blessing, it means that if you have a serious problem with your doctor (such as sexual abuse or incompetence), you have recourse to these bodies who will investigate, demand the physician be accountable, and impose penalties. As a curse, it requires physicians to answer to any number of spurious complaints from patients, most of which stem from doctor-patient encounters that the patient simply did not like. Sometimes, it's a personality conflict. You may think that these kinds of illegitimate complaints from other patients have no impact on you, but you would be wrong. Even the spurious ones are time-consuming for your doctor, taking away from both his or her time and energy for other patients, and soul-sucking. Consider what it might be like to have a doctor whose soul seems to have been sucked out. Here's an example.

I received a consult for hypnosis (my expertise in medical hypnosis put me in the position of being a consultant in this area) for a patient with what the referring physician called an "eating disorder." When the patient arrived in the office, I observed a thirty-something, clearly overweight woman whose "eating disorder" was not what I had been expecting, but nevertheless hypnosis might help her if we could identify the problem as perceived by the patient. As we were beginning the initial interview, reviewing her history, I said, "I see your weight is up. What kind of eating disorder do you have?" We then carried on with the consultation.

A few weeks later I received a formal letter from the College of Physicians and Surgeons, my provincial licensing body, informing me that a patient had filed a complaint about me. Enclosed was a lengthy letter from the patient with the "eating disorder." It seems she had complained to them that I had mentioned her weight and she found this offensive. To say I was mystified by this would be an understatement. My first thought was: if a doctor cannot comment on a clearly relevant issue like weight and health, then it's time to give up. My second thought was: why in the world did the College think it was necessary to even follow-up with such a clearly bone-headed complaint. The reason they did is because these days they will follow up on even the most specious, bogus or illegitimate complaint so that the medical profession can be perceived as transparent and accountable, regardless of the harm it causes to doctors and other patients.

Needless to say, I had to write copious letters, back and forth, defending my professional approach. Of course, in the end, the College had to admit that the complaint was baseless. However, during the period of several months (yes, several months) that it took to clear up this complaint, I was over-worked and stressed. I never doubted my position; however, I often doubted that the College would see it the same way since they had moved forward on it regardless of the nonsensical nature of the "complaint." This illustrates that although we might consider the doctor-patient relationship to be between two people, there are others who insert themselves into the equation and need to be considered.

Earlier in the book I discussed the impact of both consumer groups and pharmaceutical companies on you as a patient. It's important to remember that these groups can put pressure on medical professionals as well. When these kinds of groups inveigle themselves into the relationship you have with your primary medical provider –whether the intrusion starts with you or your doctor – it can fundamentally change the way the two of you relate to one another.

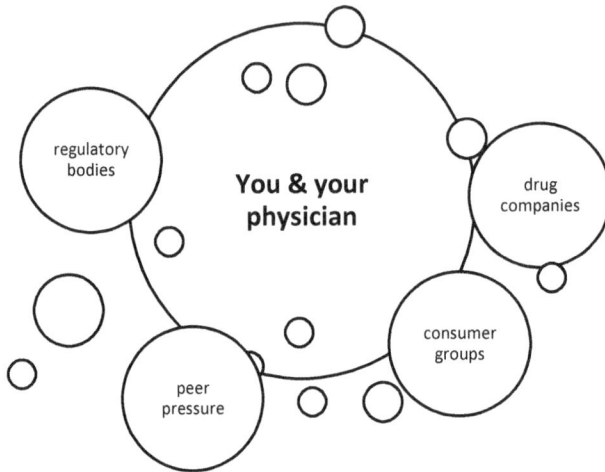

The relationship between you and your family physician or other primary healthcare provider is inherently lop-sided. When it comes to medical knowledge and access to diagnosis and treatment, your doctor clearly has more power. This puts patients in a vulnerable position. And although I mentioned that a relationship, by its very nature, is two-sided, and that doctors are only human, they are and should be held to a higher professional standard. It is the doctor who is expected to be aware of that potential vulnerability and to not exploit it. If you trust your healthcare provider, you are not likely to find yourself in the position of feeling exploited.

More attention has been given in medical education to the cultivation of interpersonal skills, communicating with patients and improving those relationships in the past two decades, but technology and computer-assisted medicine are serving to move a new wedge between doctor & patient. It's important for you to

Life is Terminal

consider these issues if you are to take a common sense approach to your relationship with your medical professional. You can only control you.

HOW IMPORTANT IS COMPATIBILITY?

Consider for a moment how you might create your bio for an online dating site. What elements of yourself would you highlight? What aspects of your personal likes and dislikes would you mention? What would you leave out? And why would you make these decisions?

I'm going to suggest that you that you make these decisions – and decisions on whether or not to respond to any interested parties in due course – based on your desire to find a compatible match. But have you really considered what it means to find someone compatible?

Someone who is compatible with you is someone who is like-minded, similar, attuned to you. It probably makes sense to you that when seeking a mate, you would search for someone compatible, with whom you could expect to get along easily, someone who shares your values. Well, common sense should also tell you that compatibility, as far as you are able to choose it, is also a hallmark of a good relationship with your primary healthcare provider.

Although there are others, I want to focus on two aspects of compatibility that I consider to be most important here: *personality* and *values*.

You may have had the experience of walking into a doctor's or nurse practitioner's office, or being approached by one of them as you lie on a hospital bed and finding yourself in a situation of disliking the person in front of you. You may know very little about them at this point, but that individual's personality does

193

not sit well with you. This can be a problem for a couple of reasons.

If you dislike your healthcare provider, or he or she dislikes you (reality check: yes, we are only human; we don't like every patient who walks into our office, and you should not expect us to), this can be a serious impediment to a good health outcome for you. One of the primary reasons for this is that it is more difficult for you to trust people you do not like (more about trust in a bit). Consequently, you are less likely to pay attention to that person, seriously hindering communication which is the key to using your healthcare to assist you in achieving your life and health goals.

Management guru Peter Drucker once said, "The most important thing in communication is hearing what isn't said." A compatible healthcare provider will be listening not only to what you are saying, but also to what you are not saying. Remember that online dating bio? What you leave out also speaks volumes.

Although it's clearly important to the physician-patient relationship that the personalities be compatible, it's not always possible, and indeed, it's sometimes not as necessary as on other occasions. First, you may not have a choice about whom you will consult. If you are an American, you may be stuck with whatever consultant is on your HMO's list. If you live in a small community, you may not have choices if you need a specialist. Or, in many places, there simply aren't enough physicians to go around for you to pick and choose. So, you have to make the best of it.

You will need all of your good communication skills at the ready to overcome a personality disconnect. Obviously, it is also the doctor's responsibility to try to overcome this, but your common sense will tell you that you cannot control someone else's responses, only your own. Thus, that's what you have to focus on.

It's up to you to find a was to communicate in this less-than-optimal situation. Remember that we all have "off" days. Don't rush to a decision based on a single encounter. It may just be the doctor's bad day.

As I mentioned above, there is a second important to aspect of compatibility – shared values. This is important and often overlooked. Let's begin by examining what I mean by values.

In general, your values are what you hold to be important in your life. And these values you hold have a direct impact on your decision-making throughout your life. Some of your personal values might include honesty, compassion, tolerance, fairness, self-reliance, civility, generosity, industriousness, courage, moderation, self-confidence, self-control etc. If you think hard enough, you may be able to identify those that you seem to hold to be the most important.

Consider the following list of values that affect your health and life journey – and your consequent health care – and check off which of these is/are important to you personally.

- ☐ Longevity
- ☐ Quality of life
- ☐ Comfort
- ☐ Cure
- ☐ Care
- ☐ Fitness
- ☐ Self-indulgence
- ☐ Honesty
- ☐ Direction
- ☐ Shared decision-making

> *When your values are clear to you, making decisions becomes easier.*
> ~ Roy E. Disney

If you are honest about assessing your own values, you can see that some of those on the above list are incompatible with one another. For example, if you value longevity – the length of life – over quality of life, this will have an enormous impact on your journey. Life-lengthening medical treatment in terminal illness, for example, will often (more often than not) result in a miserable existence, even if it does prolong your life for a period. The final outcome, however, will be no different – you will still die. Life, after all, is terminal. Further, if your primary care physician does not share this value system, you will be in conflict especially when it comes to these end-of-life situations.

These days, doctors are told to be the ones to open the discussion with patients about what is important to them. However, not all doctors will do this. In that case, common sense suggests that it will be up to you. You will need to start that discussion.

Sometimes values are dictated by an individual's religious beliefs. For example, in Canada, as a terminally ill patient, you have the right to request MAID: Medical Assistance in Dying. In other words, to choose your time of death before you suffer needlessly. Of course, as I write this, there are many legal requirements and constraints about who is eligible, but that aside, you can see that if you are making this request of a physician who has a religious belief that life must be saved at all costs – regardless of the suffering – then this person will not be amenable to assisting you. If you are terminally ill, it's important to explore your own and your physician's values surrounding death. As dramatic as this sounds, it applies equally to less dramatic situations. You still need to understand your own values and those held by others.

TRUST AND OTHER ELEMENTS OF A GREAT RELATIONSHIP

In 1994 I co-authored a book titled *When Older is Wiser: A Guide to Health Care Decisions for Older Adults and Their Families* (Toronto: Doubleday Canada). Chapter 3 focused on what my co-author and I called "Allies & Well-wishers" but its real theme centred on your relationship with your primary healthcare provider, with an emphasis on the absolute necessity of *trust*. But this trust that establishes the cornerstone of this relationship is premised on the understanding that you have to have some faith in the healthcare system in which your physician works. He or she is not isolated and cannot provide guidance to you in isolation from that system. Both of you need the system. Perhaps you can identify with the following illustration that we provided at that time.

> *"Consider what happens when the cautious traveller plans a trip. He [or she] calls his travel agent to book seats on a reputable airline. He has used this travel agent before and has some faith in her recommendations. Before leaving for the airport, he checks the weather forecast then heads out. Upon boarding the plane, he pays attention to the safety demonstration and checks the location of the exits. At some point he will have to sit back and trust that the pilots have made good decisions and have done their best. The worried passenger cannot go into the cockpit and begin to ask numerous questions about fuel and safety checks. Most passengers do not have enough basic information to do so anyway."*

This story illustrates much about our modern society. If you do not trust the engineering and construction expertise of the people who build bridges or houses, you would not cross over the bridge and could never find what you considered to be a safe place to live. If you do not have faith in the system that built your car, you would not drive it. If you do not have faith in the public health system that keeps our restaurants free from contaminants, you would never eat out. In short, you would not have any kind of a life. At some point, after your have done your due diligence, you simply have to let go of your mistrust and put some faith into your physician and the system within which he or she works if you want to use this relationship to its best advantage. This is common sense reasoning.

Influential physician and medical journal editor, the late Dr. Franz Ingelfinger who was an editor of the prestigious *New England Journal of Medicine* from 1967 to 1976 once wrote: "I do not want to be in the position of a shopper at the Casbah who negotiates and haggles with the physician about what is best. I want to believe that my physician is acting under higher moral principles and intellectual powers than a used-car salesman." However, as we said in our 1994 book, "On the other hand, Ingelfinger believes that a doctor who merely gives the patient choices and tells the patient to choose independently is shirking his or her duty to recommend a course of action after presentation of the pros and cons of the alternatives." Given the escalating influences of celebrity influencers, drug companies, consumer groups and social media in the twenty-first century, this is becoming an increasingly attractive approach for physicians. It does not result in quality care for you. Further, it does not demonstrate a physician who believes in a particular course of action or commitment to a decision. Some young, twenty-first century physicians who want to be friends with their children also carry this perspective to the doctor-patient relationship. However, neither the parent-child nor the doctor-patient relationship is a balanced one. The doctor, like the parent, should take the lead, thus earning trust.

It is well-documented that patients who trust their doctors are more likely to have good outcomes, largely because they are more likely to follow the medical advice they have sought. Study after study has demonstrated that you, the patient, will have better health and life outcomes if you trust your medical care providers. Does it not make common sense, then, for you to find a way to trust you doctor? If you truly trust your physician to help you heal, you are 30% of the way there; remember the placebo effect.

Trust, however, is not the only element that can help you to cultivate a great relationship. Others include mutual respect, honesty, and open lines of communication which lead to shared decision-making, the ultimate goal.

Mutual Respect: This seems like a no-brainer, doesn't it? If your physician does not respect you, he or she will likely not listen to and value your input into your own healthcare. If you do not respect your physician, you, too, will be prone to not listening which could have seriously detrimental effects on your life and health. You cannot have a beneficial therapeutic relationship if you lack respect for one another.

Respect starts with how you treat one another. You may think that you cannot do anything about whether or not your physician respects you as a person, but you'd be wrong. Here are some things you can do that demonstrate respect for your doctor, and that I guarantee will have a positive impact on how your doctor demonstrates respect for you:

- *Be on time for your appointments.* This shows respect for your medical practitioner's time (or other patients who are awaiting appointments). You cannot always be assured that you will get in on time, but you can be the person who is not late.

- *If you cannot make it to your appointment, call as far in advance as you can to cancel.* You'd be surprised at how many people simply do not show up. "No-shows" were a frustration for me as a doctor since I regarded this as disrespect for both me and other patients who may have been able to use that appointment slot if my office had known it would be empty. Toward the end of my practice years, I enforced a policy as follows: three missed appointments, and I fired the patient. There were too many people waiting for those slots.

- *Say please and thank-you.* These simple acts of courtesy are often a breath of fresh air in your doctor's day.

- *Present your doctor with your main reason for being there at the beginning of the appointment.* Some years ago, I was sitting in my examining room with a young man who had just gone through a litany of complaints, none of which was serious. After 40 years of practicing family medicine, I had developed a good sense of when the patient is not being completely honest. He had not come to the point. So, I said to him, "You know, this reminds me of a situation I saw last evening on *House* [the television medical drama]. He had a young patient who wasn't getting to the point. So, Dr. House got up and headed to the door at which point the patient said, 'Hey, where are you going? I'm not finished.' House replied, 'I knew when I got up to leave you would tell me why you're really here. I was just saving us both some time.'" My patient got the message and told me his real problem. A large proportion of patients get to the main complaint only as the doctor is getting up to leave. By focusing on less important aspects of your health for the appointed time, you are doing both you and your doctor a disservice. In fact, this kind of patient behaviour has led to the "one complaint per visit" policy that is currently being widely adopted by doctors and healthcare systems. And it is not popular with patients.

Open lines of communication: We've spent a lot of time earlier in this chapter discussing the importance of communication. It cannot be stressed enough that you need to keep your physician in the loop regarding any changes in your health or life status, and especially of your decisions. If you have decided, for example, to follow a course of treatment from an alternative source, it's important that you let your doctor know. It is very likely that you will want to maintain the relationship even if you're trying something else.

Honesty: This is an important element of any relationship. If you are not able to be honest with your physician, you tie his or her hands. If you omit important details related to your life and health, your doctor cannot provide you with optimum advice. Even small things can make a difference. If your doctor asks you about your eating or drinking habits, for example, don't fudge. They are important.

Shared decision-making: This is the ultimate goal. If you have a good relationship, it is more likely that you will share in the decision-making. You do not want your doctor to simply give you the pros and cons, as Dr. Ingelefinger said, and expect you to make the decision. You do not have the medical expertise to take that on independently. However, you do have the expertise about yourself, and should bring that to the table when making important health and life decisions.

ACCESS TO PHYSICIANS: PROBLEMS AND COMMON SENSE SOLUTIONS

You are probably well aware that accessing the physician or other healthcare provider you need isn't always as simple as you might think it should be. Some of these access problems have been caused by the medical profession itself: by both doctors, as well as by the medical schools from which they emanate. However, some of the problems have been caused by patients. Let's examine how these problems have evolved. I'll also offer you my opinion on how doctors and medical schools could change to improve this for your information. Then I'll offer a few common sense suggestions for you, the patient.

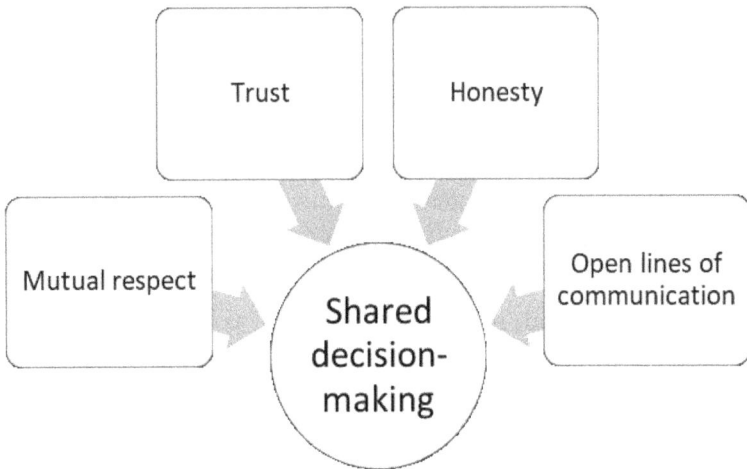

PROBLEM: PATIENTS HAVE CHANGED

It's a fact: Patients have changed. People are more uncertain these days than ever before, and this, coupled with a move toward self-centredness means that the healthcare system that served us well a half a century ago no longer works. These days, patients often need to have their beliefs reinforced by others as we've discussed earlier in the book. For example, they might encourage their friends to have a specific medical test (e.g. vitamin D level) done to reinforce their own belief that it was right for them to have it done, regardless of the fact that there is no medical indication for such a test.

Patients' expectations have also changed. People are much more focused on the "drive-through"/instant gratification kind of approach to many parts of their lives – their health care included. From my own experience, most of the complaints patients have that compel them to demand to be seen by a primary care physician immediately – urgently if you like – are issues that would resolve themselves without medical intervention within a few days or weeks. For example: muscle aches and many respiratory infections. This demand is often fed by the tsunami of information and misinformation available to everyone all the time.

Equally, medical care itself has changed. The newer paradigm of patient-centred care has resulted in complete focus on the individual. However, health funding and insurance premiums are focused on groups. The individual is unwilling to accept that whenever he or she receives medical care – whether needed or not needed – it has to be taken from someone else's care. There is only so much to go around.

Another aspect of how the delivery of primary medical care has changed has been the demands on doctors from third parties. These include such things as the increasing requirement for so-called sick notes, and the ever-present insurance claims. Compassionate doctors are more likely to develop burn-out from this, therefore are more likely to decrease their working hours.

PROBLEM: MEDICAL SCHOOLS HAVE CHANGED

It would probably come as something of a surprise to most people outside the medical and healthcare arena to know that the selection process for medical school has changed. In other words, the kind of candidates that medical schools value is different now than in the past (and I'm not referring to the fact that there are more women in medical school now). In an effort to "improve", medical schools have begun looking for more compassionate, caring individuals which seems, at first glance, like a truly good idea. However, it has had an impact on physician accessibility. These caring, compassionate people are the ones who have difficulty saying no to patients. As a result, they are unable to guide patients to accepting only the medical care that they truly need. This issue is exacerbated by the fear of either formal complaints being lodged with their colleges (the licensing bodies), or even law suits.

PROBLEM: DUBIOUS MEDICAL TREATMENT

Over the years, pharmaceutical companies have honed their skills in disease-branding, sometimes promoting dubious products to treat problems that don't need to be treated. For example: medicalizing natural human conditions such as menopause or aging. Patient groups (often – most often – funded by the very drug companies as we discussed previously) gather together to demand more tests, more drugs. But, of course, drug companies are not the only drivers of these dubious medical and healthcare treatments.

Celebrity endorsement is another problem. Celebrities, as we have discussed, push their own agendas in the media, and often vulnerable patients follow their advice often even in the face of scientific evidence to the contrary: e.g. the vaccination/autism connection still promoted by Jenny McCarthy and others despite the identification of the research as bogus.

SOLUTIONS: A FEW COMMON SENSE SUGGESTIONS

Although it's impossible for any one of us to solve the problems of access, it's worth considering solutions so that you can understand how to make the system work better for you. Here are my suggestions:

- **Patients** need to be more realistic about their health and what the collective system can reasonably be expected to provide.

- **Patients** need better skills to interpret the plethora of medical information coming at them – both unbidden and material they seek out themselves.

- **Medical schools** need to re-evaluate their methods of student selection. Too much value is placed on the subjective evaluation of individuals at interview. It could be concluded that the interviewers seek to create clones of themselves. It could further be said that medical school faculty are not the entrepreneurial, private practice types who highly value the ability of new doctors to not only treat patients, but also to manage offices and the business aspects of medical care delivery, thus improving efficiency. Doctors in the twenty-first century need both.

- **Doctors** currently in practice need to find better ways to deliver health care and more equitable ways to divide the funding made available to them in individual jurisdictions. Entrepreneurially-minded doctors and healthcare managers need to find better ways to organize the delivery of primary health care at the doctors' office level without always expecting governments to do it.

- **Doctors need to be more "response-able." They need to encourage patients to be more responsible for their own health.**

- **Drug companies** need to be more ethically responsible for their part in health care delivery.

- **Provincial disciplinary colleges** need to improve their processes. They need to move earlier to remove problem doctors and spend less time involving themselves in nuisance complaints.

- **Governments** need to find a new model to finance health care, based on what patient populations need and not on political expediency.

Although the problems seem almost insurmountable, if you understand the issues, it might make it easier to figure out how to gain access to scarce healthcare resources as you move along your life's journey.

FIGURING OUT WHAT KIND OF HEALTHCARE PROFESSIONAL MEETS YOUR NEEDS

No one can be everything to everybody. It would be helpful if you began by examining your own biases and were honest about them before making a decision about what kind of physician would meet your needs.

WHAT TO LOOK FOR IN A FAMILY PHYSICIAN (ESPECIALLY AS YOU AGE)

- A doctor who shares your value system regarding the quality versus length of life;

- A doctor who treats you with the level of respect that you require in a professional-patient relationship;

- A doctor who patiently answers all the questions that you want answered about any issue that affects your health care;

- A doctor who is able to be honest about any limitations he or she might have regarding your wishes for your future care;

- A doctor who stays actively involved in your care even if you require referral to a specialist of one kind or another.

[Source: Patricia Parsons & Arthur Parsons. *When Older is Wiser: A Guide to Health Care Decisions for Older Adults and their Families.* Toronto, Doubleday, 1994, p. 43.]

But what about those situations when you have little choice about your physician?

One of the approaches you can take is to become your own main care-giver using your doctor for access to things you cannot access yourself: tests, treatments, prescriptions – let the physician or other healthcare provide be your conduit. You may not have your ideal doctor, but you can use this individual to access specialists who may better suit your needs.

Inevitably, though, there will be times when you will come into conflict with even the most compatible care giver. From a physician's point of view, there is probably one thing that will initiate a conflict more than any other: when a patient refuses to follow the advice that he or she has sought. The medical profession refers to this as "the non-compliant patient."

After you have consulted with a medical expert, undergone tests, had all of your questions answered and been provided with a recommended course of action, your refusal to follow advice and yet continue to appear for further consultation will generally cause a conflict in your relationship. Obviously, the way to avoid this is to have those open lines of communication, share in the decision-making, and follow the *mutually agreed upon* course of action. Any other approach would be nonsensical.

Your relationship with your primary medical care provider will be very important as you get closer and closer to that terminus on your life's journey. Knowing how to navigate these relationships, and applying some common sense will serve to smooth the path ahead.

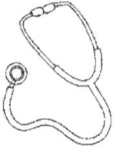

KEYS TO RELATING WELL TO YOUR PHYSICIAN (AND OTHER HEALTH PROFESSIONALS)

☑ Take time to consider the human-ness of your physician rather than thinking about him or her as super-human.

☑ Seek healthcare providers who are compatible with you.

☑ Explore your healthcare providers' values to determine your compatibility.

☑ Examine the extent to which you trust your doctor, and take steps to improve it.

☑ Treat your doctor with the level of respect that you expect in return.

☑ Be honest.

☑ Keep the lines of communication open.

☑ Move toward the goal of shared decision-making.

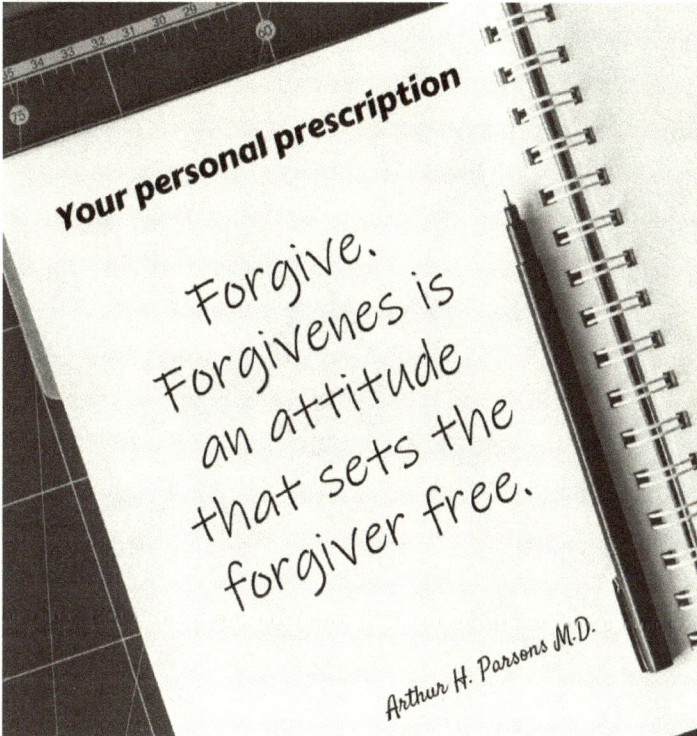

Your personal prescription

Forgive.
Forgivenes is
an attitude
that sets the
forgiver free.

Arthur H. Parsons M.D.

Parsons

CHAPTER ELEVEN

COMMON SENSE IN ACTION: TAKING RESPONSIBILITY

*"The secret of health for both mind and body is not
to mourn for the past, not to worry about the future,
or to anticipate troubles, but to live in the present moment
wisely and earnestly."*
~ The Buddha

WAY BACK AT THE BEGINNING of this book, I suggested to you that being responsible is actually the key to our common sense. Before I finish the common sense guide, it's important that you understand that taking responsibility is the most important way you can put common sense into action.

There is one hard truth of life that should be clear to you by this point in our discussion: You are responsible for your own health and happiness. This does, however, not mean that everything that happens to you is your fault – use some common sense – but it does mean that your happiness is an inside job, and how you respond to your life as it unfolds will affect that. Illness may not always be under your control, but how you frame your personal story about it and how you respond to what happens to you certainly are under your control and will have an impact on your journey.

This is not just my opinion. Over the past two decades, there has been a lot written in the self-help arena on the topic of *personal*

211

responsibility. One of the earliest (and subsequently most popular) books on the topic was written in 1997 by American psychotherapist Nathaniel Branden. He suggests that "...an attitude of self-responsibility must be generated from within the individual. It cannot be 'given' from the outside..." So, it does not matter what I or anyone else tries to make you feel about the importance of taking personal responsibility, you have to work to cultivate it within yourself. This is perhaps the most important common sense approach to having a good journey to the end of life.

Being responsible, however, is often combined with the notion of being an "adult." Do you really know what an adult is, though? Perhaps we should begin our discussion there – with understanding the concept of responsible adulthood.

WHAT IT MEANS TO BE A RESPONSIBLE *ADULT*

What does it really mean to be an adult? It's likely that you haven't given this much conscious thought. If you are an older adult, you may, from time to time, have looked at a young adult and said (maybe to yourself unless it was one of your own children), "Grow up," or "Act like an adult..." But what do you really mean by that? What does "acting like an adult" look like?

Growing up is such a barbarous business, full of inconvenience... and pimples. ~ J.M. Barrie (from Peter Pan)

You have a picture in your head of what you personally believe to be what adult behaviour looks like. But it's important if we're going to define personal responsibility – which is something that can really only reasonably be expected of an adult, that we have a shared understanding of those behaviours.

I'm sure we all know people over 30, or even over 40, whose age suggests to us that they are, or at least ought to be adults, yet we look at them and think, "Peter Pan." Remember him? The man-child who never grew up? The child who always stayed a child? Notwithstanding the Peter Pans around you, are you really certain that *you* are, indeed, an adult?

According to psychologist Dr. Robert Firestone, adults approach life in a particular way, and these become the hallmarks for identifying adults versus those who have not matured into adulthood as yet. He identifies the following five characteristics by which we recognize adults:

1. rationality, meaning that a true adult can differentiate between emotions and intellect;

2. the ability to formulate goals and take actions that will get you there;

3. the ability to ensure that equality is the hallmark of your personal relationships;

4. taking an active approach to life rather than passively maintaining the victim mentality; and,

5. the ability to be open to criticism without defensiveness.

When you think about these, aren't these among the common sense approaches to life that we've been talking about for the past ten chapters?

I'm going to suggest to you that being a mature adult (by which I do not mean "senior") means recognizing that you are responsible for your own life – the life that results from the choices you make.

The truth is that you are responsible for all the good choices that you have made. You are equally responsible for all of the bad choices you have made. When you say 'no' to one thing, you are saying 'yes' to another, and vice versa.

For example, at some point in your life you chose to be a smoker or to be a non-smoker. Let's say you chose to take that first cigarette, then carried the habit on from there. Go ahead and argue that you had no choice – you were in a situation that made the choice impossible. Bullsh*t. You had a choice in that moment; you always have a choice. Either you made a good one or you made a bad one. And remember, making no choice is also a choice. If you said yes to smoking, then you said no to the healthy lungs and heart – not to mention better skin – that you could otherwise have had. Choosing one path over another one, has consequences.

RESPONSIBILITY AND ACCOUNTABILITY

Up until this point in our discussion, I've used the terms "adult" and "responsible adult" more or less synonymously. But what does the qualifier *responsible* really mean? And how does that relate to the concept of being *accountable*? Let's start with responsibility.

Conventional definitions suggest that to be responsible is to have an obligation to do something. If you are responsible for the coffee in your lunch room at the office, you have an obligation to ensure that there is coffee there when people want or need it. Being responsible also means to *have control over someone or some thing*. As a parent you are responsible for your children's care and feeding: you have control over it. It can also mean that you are *the cause of something*. If you caused a car accident by texting while driving, you are responsible for it. So, *being responsible relates to you having obligations, control and accountability*. Accountability is accepting responsibility and being answerable. It also means being honest with yourself. In our search for a common sense approach to your health and life journey, it only makes sense that you would accept that you are responsible – and accountable to yourself. Taking responsibility means taking ownership. And if you don't own your own life and health, who does? Perhaps it's time to listen to yourself. You cannot hear yourself, though, until you say, "I am responsible."

On the following page I've presented a proposal for you. It incorporates a number of recommendations for moving in the direction of being truly responsible for your own life and health.

In simple terms, being responsible for your life choices means being *response-able*, being *able to respond*, rather than to react or cop out and play the victim card. And there is a big difference between a reaction and a response.

Consider the following scenario: You are sitting across from your family doctor who has just told you the results of a diagnostic test you underwent the previous week. You are a married, sexually monogamous adult who has just been told you have hepatitis B. You know that the only ways you can contract hep B are through contaminated needles (you're not a junkie, or even a healthcare worker who could have been accidentally stuck by a contaminated needle), having it passed from mother to child (a non-starter in your case), or sexual relations. Do you immediately react to this news, or do you respond?

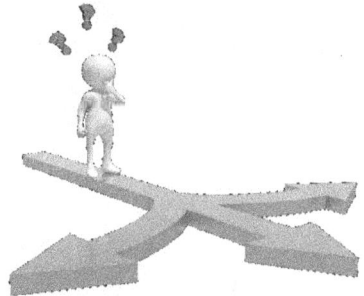

RESPONSIBILITY PROPOSAL

R •*Respect* yourself, *read* widely, do your *research*.

E •*Expect* the best but be prepared for the unexpected.

S •*Say* the right thing. Always.

P •Practice shifting your *paradigm* whenever necessary.

O •Be *open* to ideas different from your own.

N •Never say *never.*

S •Consider that *self-help* means to help yourself.

I •"*If* it's to be, it's up to me."

B •*Believe* in yourself.

L •Consider the *long-term effects* of your actions.

E •*Educate* yourself, and *embrace* yourself.

Do you immediately begin ranting and raving about your spouse who must have been unfaithful to you while your doctor sits in front of you watching you disembowel your relationship? Or do you ask some pertinent questions, begin to educate yourself about this disease, think about the answers, consider what this might (or might not) mean for your health and your relationship, then deal with your immediate health problem knowing that you will likely have to have an uncomfortable conversation with your spouse? The way you act in reply to this news sets the stage for being able to take control and deal with the consequences of the news, or letting it control you. You can react, as in the first approach, or respond, as in the second.

According to psychologist, Dr. Matt James, "A reaction is instant. It's driven by the beliefs, biases, and prejudices of the unconscious mind…A response…usually comes more slowly…based on information from both the conscious mind and unconscious mind… It weighs the long-term effects." Wouldn't you like to think that you are also employing your conscious thought processes and the immediate situation in addition to your biases and preformed ideas? In an emotionally charged situation it's often difficult to consider the long-term effects, but it's worth cultivating the ability to respond rather than to react. Because there are consequences. Remember, if you identify as a "victim" you have given up control to someone else. You have chosen not to be response-able. Give control up to circumstances or an aggressor and you will always be controlled by circumstances or someone else.

During my internship, in the last year of medical school, my wife and I were driving across Newfoundland to spend a month interning in St. John's. Outside Stephenville a car pulled onto the highway in front of me forcing us through a guard rail and down an embankment. I suffered a broken nose and facial injuries and my wife a fractured spine. I blamed the other driver for years and spent time on insurance claims.

Later in life when I took the idea of responsibility to heart, I analyzed the day to see what part I played in this event. I realized that at breakfast, several hours before the accident, a server was very slow and incompetent, in my view. I paid and we left early in a huff. What I later realized was that this person was trying to slow me down so I would not be there when the other driver pulled onto the highway. Thus, I changed my story and it is the one I have been telling ever since.

THERE ARE CONSEQUENCES: OR GETTING OUT OF YOUR OWN WAY

What happens to you is what happens to you, whether you take control of it and influence the direction you're going in life, or you don't. If you choose to take the latter approach – refusing to take responsibility for your adult actions – there are consequences. The proximate or short-term consequences may not be as life-altering as the long-term, and therefore less imminent, consequences can be. This is one of the short-sighted reasons that people sometimes do not take responsibility. But it will catch up with you sooner or later.

> *All human sin seems so much worse in its consequences than in its intentions.* ~ Reinhold Niebuhr

There are so many other people and things you can blame for your circumstances at any given time, aren't there? You can blame your parents, spouse, siblings, boss, or friends. You can blame your personal economic circumstances or the state of the society in which you live. But blaming any of these external sources isn't going to change a single thing in your life. As long as you abdicate personal responsibility with the mantra, "It's not my fault," then you will always be where you are. You will not be able to get out of your own way. And *you need to get out of your own way.* If *you* take responsibility you may find it is easier to forgive yourself since you are aware of all the extenuating circumstances, a situation that cannot happen if you place the responsibility (or blame) on someone else even though that person may have unknown reasons for their actions. After all, forgiveness is and act that sets the forgiver free. *Isn't that freedom what we all desire?*

As said I said before, maybe it was Sigmund Freud, perhaps Albert Einstein, or it may even have been Mark Twain (although the best evidence suggests it was American novelist Rita Mae Brown in 1983 who first said it), but the definition of insanity as doing the same thing over and over and expecting different results, regardless of its provenance, is worth considering. Perhaps it's not really insanity, but it is certainly a misguided way to live your life.

Consider this. You have just been diagnosed with diabetes. Your doctor and dietitian have spent some quality time working through a regimen with you: medication, exercise, diet. You return to the doctor only to discover that your blood sugar is still unstable. If you were to be honest with the doctor, you would just say it: you expected that the pills alone would work. You have not changed the way you are eating. You like your daily chocolate bars. You are continuing the same behaviour and expecting different results. Neither your doctor nor the dietitian ever suggested that the pills alone would work: *your behaviour would have to change*. You can see how this would not serve you well. So, there are consequences to your choices.

Well-known American author Dr. Norman Cousins was one of the pioneers of research on the effects of emotions on human health and illness, and author of the bestselling classic *Anatomy of an Illness*. He once said, "A human being fashions his consequences as surely as he fashions his goods or his dwelling. Nothing that he says, thinks or does is without consequence." This is as true in your life journey and health decisions as it is in your everyday life.

ARE YOU REALLY RESPONSIBLE FOR EVERYTHING THAT HAPPENS TO YOUR HEALTH?

I'm sure that by now you are wondering, "Am I really responsible for everything that happens to me…to my health?" "Does he think I'm responsible for my own illness?" "Am I really to blame for my diagnosis?" Perhaps you are even angry at the thought that this might be true. Let's step back for a moment and apply some common sense: of course not. Of course, in general, you are not directly responsible for every bad thing (or every good thing) that happens to you. That is a nonsensical way to approach

> *While we are free to choose our actions, we are not free to choose the consequences of our actions.*
> ~ Stephen R. Covey

life and health, including any given diagnosis. But every decision you make certainly does have an impact on what follows. On the other hand, there is certainly ample research data for us to conclude that lifestyle factors over which you have complete control, certainly do have an impact on your health and the quality of your life. This is the place where you can begin to make those choices after weighing the consequences.

According to American medical researcher Dr. David Resnik writing in the *Journal of Medical Ethics*, "Six of the 10 leading factors contributing to the global burden of disease are lifestyle related: unsafe sex, high blood pressure, tobacco use, alcohol use, high cholesterol and obesity." (His conclusion was drawn from data from the World Health Organization.) Further, according to the annual report on *The State of Obesity* (this report series is a collaborative project of the Trust for America's Health and the Robert Wood Johnson Foundation) …

> *"Obesity is one of the biggest drivers of preventable chronic diseases and healthcare costs in the United States. Currently, estimates for*

these costs range from $147 billion to nearly $210 billion per year. In addition, obesity is associated with job absenteeism, costing approximately $4.3 billion annually and with lower productivity while at work, costing employers $506 per obese worker per year."

With this in mind as an illustration, consider Dr. Resnik's further thoughts on these lifestyle conditions. Since your lifestyle *choices* that have a negative impact on your personal health also have a negative impact on society, Dr. Resnick wonders if you should not be held morally responsible for your poor decisions. After all, this negative impact includes creating a burden on scarce resources as well as contributing to an economic burden on society. In other words, he is asking whether or not you should be able to have equal access to scarce healthcare resources beside others whose illnesses were less a matter of choice. Should the person with alcohol-related liver failure be given the same access to a liver for transplantation as the person whose liver failure was a result of an overwhelming infection of unknown origin? These are ethical dilemmas related to the allocation of scarce medical resources. This could ultimately be one of the consequences you may have to face as a consequence of your choices. But what about those illnesses that appear to be more a matter of fate or poor luck or simply aging? Can you be held responsible for those?

If you apply common sense to this question, you realize that it would be absurd to consider everyone responsible for every single thing that happens in life. That being said, as I have said (and it's worth repeating) **you most assuredly are responsible for how you respond to these situations.** Reconsider our discussion earlier in this chapter about the difference between a *response* and a *reaction*, then consider the consequences of each of them.

DON'T WASTE YOUR TIME: IT'S FINITE

You do not have "all the time in the world." You are not going to live forever. Your life, just like the lives of everyone else in your life and on this planet, is terminal; even the planet itself will die in time. Get this through your head and everything changes.

You *are* going to die some day. Despite fake news, alternative facts, and constant public lies, no one can deny this simple fact. Now that you have accepted this, how are you going to live the life

This is your life. You are responsible for it. You will not live forever. Don't wait.
~ Natalie Goldberg

you have left? You'll notice that I purposely did not ask you how you will spend the "time" you have left. This is because the relative time may be long or short, or it may seem long or short, depending on how you decide to live. You may have many years, of only a few days or hours. No one knows.

A child may die having lived a good life. An old person may die never having lived at all. How do you define "living"? If you let it be so, it could simply be time spent on earth, or it could be experiences linked together by happiness or good thoughts. Because, in the end, your life is the story you tell yourself, connecting events that you create or that happen to you. Thus, it doesn't matter if you believe that you have free will or that your life is pre-determined: you make up the story you tell yourself, and if you don't like it, make up another one that you do like.

It was always an important opportunity for me to help a patient who arrived in my medical office with a tale of woe. This tale is the story the patient had told him or herself. I would say to this patient, "I can spin the same facts you've just presented into another story, and if you accept this new version and make it yours, it will make you feel better." Then I would offer my version of the story. Sometimes the patient would laugh; occasionally the patient would accept it, but often not. Usually, the patient's tale served his or her needs better for a variety of reasons. The patient saw no reason to change. I have always maintained that if patients believed a different version of their stories, that story had the power to change them.

After forty-five years of seeing patients in my office day after day, there is one thing I know for sure: people would rather feel anger or guilt than feel helpless. If you take responsibility for your own health and life, you are no longer helpless. That feeling evaporates. As Eleanor Roosevelt once said, "In the long run, we shape our lives, and we shape ourselves. The process never ends until we die. And the choices we make are ultimately our own responsibility."

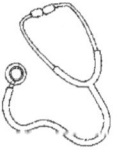

THE KEY TO UNDERSTANDING THAT LIFE IS TERMINAL

Time is the best teacher.
Unfortunately, it kills all its students.

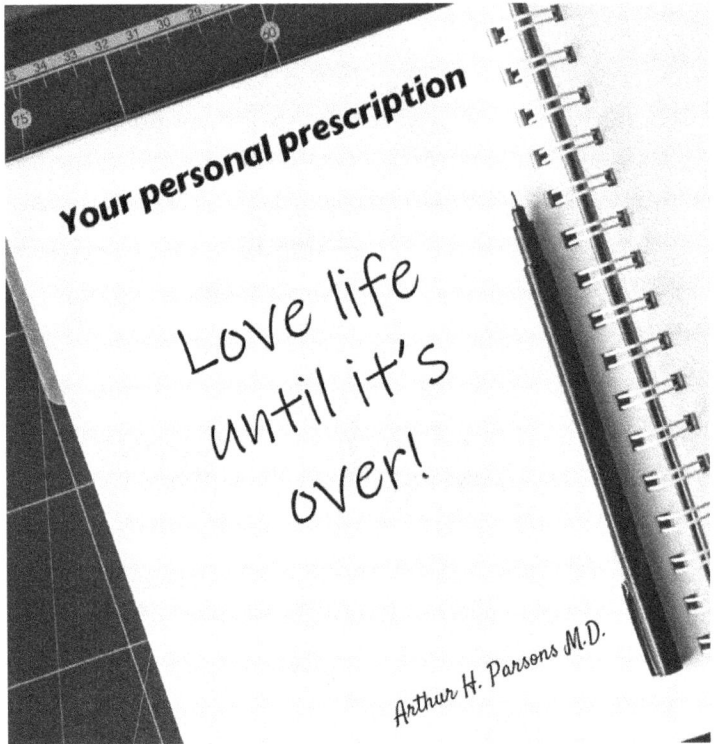

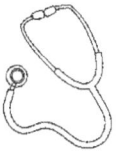

BACK IN THE OFFICE...ONE LAST TIME

DR. PETE KOWALSKI STOOD OUTSIDE the building where his office occupied the second floor. He gazed up at the window where he had looked out every working day for the past thirty-five years. He was remembering his very first day on the job, when he had contemplated his name on the door under the names of two other doctors who would become important mentors and colleagues. Dr. Kramer had long since retired, and Dr. Fontaine had retired three years ago. Now it was his turn. The two other names on the door these days were of two new, young colleagues who brought a breath of fresh air to the practice, and yet seemed to have such a different view of the world. He sighed.

He waved to the new receptionist as he walked toward his private office in the rear. He could see two of his long-time patients were already in the waiting room, looking at him anxiously as he smiled in acknowledgement. They'll be fine, he thought, despite the fact he knew that their anxiety about their future family physician prospects was well founded: he had been unable to secure a new doctor to take over his practice. It seemed that his patient roster and workload were too great for many of the newly minted family physicians who valued work-life balance over all else. How times had changed.

Despite it being his final day in the office, the day was much like any other. His very last patient of the day told him he had specifically requested this final slot—he wanted to be Pete's very last patient. Pete was glad since this patient was one who always left him with a feeling of gratitude for having the privilege of being a doctor. Because, deep in his heart, and despite the many challenges of practicing medicine these days, it *was* a privilege, and Pete knew it.

After the patient left, Pete was alone, sitting at his desk, contemplating scooping up the final vestiges of his belongings to carry on with the next chapter of his life. But he was thinking, *What have I learned?*

First, he considered the one big conundrum he had never been able to figure out: *Why is it that so many people seem to believe that life, whatever it has deteriorated to, has to be maintained indefinitely no matter the cost: money, people, resources, psychological stress?* To this question, he had no answer. But he had learned a few things.

He knew that many of his patients had held onto their suffering for a variety of reasons, one of the most insidious had been to gain attention of one sort or another. Sometimes it was attention from him, but often it was attention from friends and family. It was sad.

He had also learned, sometimes the hard way, that everyone has a shadow side that they usually try to suppress. He now knew that you had to own that shadow side if you wanted to heal.

In the end he knew that if there was one thing he could have taught his patients it was this: *Take your life in your hands and live it as if it matters.*

"Yes," he said out loud to himself, "that's just what I'll do. Onward!" Because, after all, life is terminal.

The End

EPILOGUE

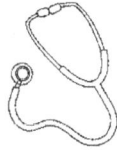

WHY I WROTE THIS BOOK

WHEN I LOOK BACK ON MY CHILDHOOD, I realize that I was always introspective, reflective and perhaps a bit brooding. When I was very young I asked a lot of questions, mostly "why's". I was constantly asking questions like, "Why can't I fly?" or, "When I close my eyes, does the world get dark?" My mother answered the second question easily, but had more of a problem with the first one. The years marched onward and I grew up, eventually entering that strange world of the teenager when attitudes change. I was opinionated and angry, leaving home at seventeen to study science at university, and it was during my second year that everything changed. Looking back, I now realize that this change in me was influenced by a single person.

The person who shaped that change in me was my sophomore English professor. A run-of-the-mill university English course, it was unlike some of the more esoteric subjects that college English courses seem to focus on these days. For me, though, it wasn't the content of the course that was important: it was the way this professor taught.

This professor had a framework he called the *theory of the creative eye* that I seized on, soon learning that the "eye" he referred to also meant "I". Through his theory he suggested that the observer, not liking the world he or she is living in, looks in a mirror and creates a world of ideas, then lives in that world among these new ideas. In a mirror image, right is left and left is right, the image is reversed. If we look at another mirror image of the mirror image, things are again the "right way around." The only way we can then see the original reality is to look at that mirror image of the mirror image, thus returning to reality. The theory further suggested, could best be done through art, stage plays in particular where, like a mirror, stage left is on the right of the audience. After being exposed to this idea, I began questioning the world that we commonly accept as reality. And often the answers I perceived were unexpected.

Many years later I found myself standing in a bookstore in Portland, Maine. I was quietly examining a rack of books when a man, whom I did not know and had not noticed standing near me, said, "I think that you would like this one if you can get past the religious bit," as he pointed to a book titled *The Power of Your Subconscious Mind* by Joseph Murphy, a name with which I was unfamiliar at the time.

For some reason, I took the stranger's advice and bought the book. I devoured the pages finding that I wanted to read more by the author, but could not find his work anywhere. (There was only a handful of bookstores where I lived at the time, and no online behemoth book sellers). I have since come to know Joseph Murphy as a prolific Irish-American author with a Ph.D. and a Doctor of Divinity who wrote widely on affirmative thinking and the power of your mind until his death in 1981.

Some time after reading this book, and wanting more, I found myself doing something that was out of character for me. One weekend, my family wanted to go to a garage sale, so I went along. Garage sales were not my "thing." To my amazement, I happened upon three more books by Joseph Murphy. These three books led me to a steady stream of other related books and authors.

Somewhere along this journey through ideas, I stumbled upon a single idea that resonated with me and that I have thus never forgotten: "Open a book, any book, any page and there you will find the answers you need." And so, I did.

At this time, I was a practising physician with a busy family medicine practice, deeply entrenched in the science of medicine, so I found this concept difficult to comprehend. However, I now recognize the concept works because you really do already have the answer within you, and if you read words on a page (or an e-reader) you can interpret them in any way you want to give you the answer that you need, and already know. The truth is that you will often accept that answer because you believe it came from outside you, from a superior source, even though it probably didn't. The *I Ching* – the ancient Chinese divination system – likely works in the same way, providing vague answers that you can interpret in many ways. We seldom trust ourselves, but we should. If we did trust our innate intelligence and were honest with ourselves, we would realize that we usually already know the answer if we are willing to hear it.

At some point along my own path I also came to believe that before we are born and shortly thereafter, we each intuitively feel at one with the universe. Then over the years, we begin to develop boundaries and to define ourselves. We see something we don't like and say, "I'm not like that," or think, "I am this." This is the point at which my old English professor would say we enter the mirror world. The truth is that we still are whole, and the thing that we arbitrarily "cut off" from ourselves is what has been described by psychologists as our "shadow side." It is always there whether we allow ourselves to recognize it or not. We might even consciously deny it, sometimes very strongly. Life, however we might wish it to be, is not black *or* white; light *or* dark; good *or* evil. It is black *and* white; light *and* dark; good *and* evil. It is all of it.

When we accept something – a single something – to be true, we deny its opposite. It is this opposite, our shadow, that controls most people. If we recognize it and accept it, we have gone a long way toward health and happiness. And there are ways to recognize and accept our shadows.

When I was in grade school I got into a fight with a friend as my classmates watched. After it was over a classmate who had witnessed the spectacle said this: "I would not want to get into a fight with you because you looked as if you could kill him." So, I guess I have always had a killer instinct in addition to my predisposition as a healer. Two opposites. I have never really rejected that killer instinct, since this part of who I am protected me from bullies, but I never accepted him, either, or allowed him to take control. He is my shadow, but since I acknowledge him, he is not an unconscious part of me.

If you don't like someone, or one of that individual's personal characteristics, you are probably seeing your own unconscious or unacknowledged shadow that you have projected onto that person. Thus, how you relate to this person becomes your approach to dealing with your own shadow side. The problem is that you can never really accept your own shadow if you see it only in someone else. However, it is another example of accepting responsibility. Accepting your own shadow will improve your relationship with the other individual.

Besides "works of art" one of the ways we can begin to learn about ourselves and accept all facets of who we are is through hypnotic techniques. My interest goes back many years. As a young child, I was an avid comic book fan. But beyond the stories contained in the comics, I was fascinated by the advertisements on the back covers. Among those ads were enticing offers for learning hypnosis, or "mind control" as it was described. After I graduated from medical school and had been practising for ten years, I had an opportunity to learn to do "medical hypnosis" which I subsequently used regularly as a part of what I offered to patients until I retired. Even now, I still use self-hypnosis for things like relaxation. What's even more interesting about this is that some of the techniques used in hypnosis are used regularly in advertising which says a lot about its power to change minds.

Over the years, I took advantage of opportunities to learn more about hypnosis and to deepen my understanding of its processes and uses. Through continuing education programs offered by hypnosis societies such as Canadian Society of Clinical Hypnosis, I was exposed to a variety of approaches and theories. One in particular interested me. I had the opportunity to hear Dr. Bruce Lipton, an American developmental biologist and author of the book *The Biology of Belief* speak at a conference. You'll recall I referenced his work in the preceding pages. I found his approach provided me with a helpful explanation of the connection between mind and body. I recommend his work to anyone interested in this topic.

Greek philosopher Heraclitus wrote, "Nothing endures but change." He was so right. Even a river that appears to be still has a constant flow. We need to embrace change and enjoy it. Many – if not most – people resist change, spending most of their lives clinging to relationships, things or ideas. Rather than resisting the inevitable process of change, we should go with the flow and stop paddling upstream in order to attempt to stand still. This constant struggle against change is very tiring and energy-consuming, and can play a part in ill health.

One other important concept that has become important to me through the years is the notion that words and language can have such a profound effect. My perspective on this has been influenced largely by my education and experience in the area of hypnotherapy.

Over the years, I have been fascinated by three words that are often inscribed on Christmas cards. These words are *peace, love and joy*. During periods of meditation and self-hypnosis, I have been able to access these states to the point where merely saying each of these words while relaxing produces each of these states. I began to wonder how I could explain this to other people so they could do the same. I came up with a BAG to contain these states.

B: BE IN THE MOMENT. Stop thinking, stop analysing and simply be. My wife once gave me a plaque with the following words inscribed on it: "Be still and know that I am."

A: ACCEPT AND APPRECIATE. Accept the moment and circumstances for what they are. Stop fighting or wanting it to be other than it is. Appreciate the moment. If you find it difficult to do that, appreciate the moment by adding value to it. Reframe it. You can always appreciate something by realizing that whatever it is, it could be worse.

G: EXPRESS GRATITUDE. Give thanks to the universe for the moment and what it brings. In our western culture where many people have so much, few seem happy with what they have, always wanting more. Gratitude seems to be a lost concept. Being thankful for whatever you have been given is very powerful. If you can't be grateful, tell yourself a different story about the circumstances that allows you to feel grateful. "At least I'm alive." The actual feeling of thanks is the state you are trying to achieve. Imagine what it would feel like to realize that you just survived a serious accident, or your doctor just told you that a terminal illness has disappeared. Experience that feeling in your thoughts, but especially in that relaxed, total body feeling of letting go.

When you do all of this, you are at *peace*. In this peace you can express unconditional *love*. When you express that love, you will experience *joy*.

Notice that these states are not intellectual, or in thought only. They constitute a total body experience: A true feeling of being One.

When I was in my early thirties, I began experiencing an irregular heartbeat. Concluding that it was the result of stress, I took a vacation. Just as I had hoped, the irregular beats stopped, so I decided to take things a bit easier. This worked for a while, however, in spite of my newly relaxed lifestyle, the irregularities came back. I finally realized that the irregularities occurred when I was not in balance, and I used their presence or absence to that define my balance point. I soon learned that this point was a moving target, and balance a dance. I'm still working on understanding the dance and learning new steps.

Many of these are ideas that have come to shape my life have helped me to guide patients along their health and life journeys and have ultimately shaped this book. My wife (and co-author) and I began to think about writing this book at the turn of the millennium in 2000. It had several false starts, and we put it away. When I retired from my full-time medical practice in 2014, I relaxed. We traveled quite a lot for several years, and my heartbeat irregularities stayed away. About three years after retirement and increased relaxation, this irregular heart rhythm returned. I tried all my "tricks" to try to control it, but nothing seemed to be working. I did a little introspective examination and asked myself, "Why?" I got the impression that I was not supposed to retire from everything. Then I asked, "What am I supposed to do?" This book returned to my consciousness, and I now had another purpose. The heart irregularity subsided as I worked on it, and will likely lead me to other paths in the future. I hope you have enjoyed the results, or at least the book has made you think. Perhaps it will help you with your never-ending dance of balance.

*~ **Arthur H. Parsons*** B.Sc., M.D., Toronto, June, 2019

Parsons

LIFE IS TERMINAL: SOURCES

J. Alcock. We are our beliefs. *Psychology Today* online. February 14, 2018. https://www.psychologytoday.com/ca/blog/belief/201802/we-are-our-beliefs

T. Armstrong. Multiple intelligences. *American Institute for Learning and Human Development*. http://www.institute4learning.com/resources/articles/multiple-intelligences/

M. Borins. *A doctor's guide to alternative medicine: What works, what doesn't, and why*. 2014. Helena, Montana: Lyons Press.

N. Branden. *Taking responsibility: Self-reliance and the accountable life*. 1997. New York: Fireside, p. 191.

H. Braude. *Intuition in medicine: A philosophical defense of clinical reasoning*. 2012. Chicago: University of Chicago Press.

A. Brenner. 8 things the most toxic people in your life have in common. *Psychology Today* online. August 29, 2016. https://www.psychologytoday.com/ca/blog/in-flux/201608/8-things-the-most-toxic-people-in-your-life-have-in-common

O. Burkeman. *The antidote: Happiness for people who can't stand positive thinking*. New York: Penguin Books ltd., 2012.

D. Chopra in C. Pert. *Molecules of emotion: The science behind mind-body medicine*. New York: Touchstone, 1997.

F. Cholle. *The Intuitive Compass: Why the best decisions balance reason and instinct*. 2011. Jossey-Bass.

F. Cholle. What is intuition, and how do we use it? *Psychology Today*. August 31, 2011.
https://www.psychologytoday.com/ca/blog/the-intuitive-compass/201108/what-is-intuition-and-how-do-we-use-it

J. Coupland. (2003). Small talk: Social functions. *Research on Language and Social Interaction*. 36. pp. 1-6.

K. Crowe. Following the money between patient groups and Big Pharma. *CBC News* online. March 21, 2018.
https://www.cbc.ca/news/health/second-opinion-patient-advocacy-pharmaceutical-industry-funding-drug-prices-1.4539271

H. Dunn. High-level wellness for man and society. *American Journal of Public Health*. Vol. 49, No. 6, June, 1959, pp. 786-792.
https://www.ncbi.nlm.nih.gov/pmc/articles/PMC1372807/?page=1

R. Firestone. Six aspects of being an adult. *Psychology Today*. June 24, 2013.
https://www.psychologytoday.com/ca/blog/the-human-experience/201306/six-aspects-being-adult

M. Friedman & R. Rosenman. Association of specific overt behaviour pattern with blood and cardiovascular findings. *Journal of the American Medical Association*, Vol. 169, March 21, 1959, pp. 1286-1296.

M. Friedman & R. Rosenman and others. The relationship of behaviour pattern A to the state of the coronary vasculature: A study of 51 autopsy subjects. *American Journal of Medicine*. Vol. 44, April, 1968, pp. 525-537.

M. Gallucci. Here are just a few of the problematic controversies of 'The Dr. Oz Show' *Mashable*. September 15, 2016.

https://mashable.com/2016/09/15/donald-trump-health-dr-oz/#OEZDtPcuwiqY

B. Hendrick. Survey shows Americans trust their doctors. *WebMD*. December 3, 2010. https://www.webmd.com/a-to-z-guides/news/20101203/survey-shows-americans-trust-their-doctors#1

R. Holiday. 10 strategies for turning obstacles into opportunities. *Meditations on Strategy and Life*. https://ryanholiday.net/10-strategies-for-turning-obstacles-into-opportunities/

Ipsos Research. Canadians trust their doctors to make the right choice… July 13, 2016. https://www.ipsos.com/en-ca/news-polls/canadians-trust-their-doctors-make-right-choice-patients-and-doctors-believe-strongly-cost-should

M. James. React vs respond: What's the difference? *Psychology Today*. September 1, 2016. https://www.psychologytoday.com/ca/blog/focus-forgiveness/201609/react-vs-respond

D. Khullar. Do you trust the medical profession? *New York Times*. January 23, 2018. https://www.nytimes.com/2018/01/23/upshot/do-you-trust-the-medical-profession.html

L. Lacey. 'Pinkwashing' and the dark side of breast-cancer philanthropy. *The Globe and Mail*. February 3, 2012. https://www.theglobeandmail.com/arts/film/pinkwashing-and-the-dark-side-of-breast-cancer-philanthropy/article543081/

C. Lieberman. How self-care became so much work. *Harvard Business Review*. August 10, 2018. https://hbr.org/2018/08/how-self-care-became-so-much-work

B. Lipton. *The biology of belief: Unleashing the power of unconsciousness, matter and miracles*. 2005. Mountain of Love/Elite.

M. McCoy, Ph.D., M. Carniol, M.B.A., K. Chockley, B.A., and others. Conflicts of interest for patient-advocacy organizations. *New England Journal of Medicine*. Vol. 376, March 2, 2017, pp. 880-885. https://www.nejm.org/doi/full/10.1056/NEJMsr1610625

Merriam-Webster Dictionary online. *Self-help*. https://www.merriam-webster.com/dictionary/self-help

National Center for Complementary and Integrative Health (Us Department of Health & Human Services). Finding and evaluating online resources. https://nccih.nih.gov/health/webresources

G. Oettingen and others. Pleasure now, pain later: Positive fantasies about the future predict symptoms of depression. *Psychological Science*. Vol. 27; No. 3, pp. 345-353, January 29, 2016. https://journals.sagepub.com/doi/abs/10.1177/0956797615620783

L. O'Leary and P. Velasco. The industry of wellness, by the numbers. *Marketplace*. January 4, 2018. https://www.marketplace.org/2018/01/04/world/wellness-craze-numbers

P. Parsons and A Parsons. *When older is wiser: A guide to healthcare decisions for older adults and their families*. 1994. Toronto: Doubleday Canada.

D. Resnik. Responsibility for health: personal, social, and environmental. *Journal of Medical Ethics*. August, 2007; 33(8): 444–445.

https://www.ncbi.nlm.nih.gov/pmc/articles/PMC2598168/

W. Sheldon. What Is intellect? Part one. *Philosophy East and West.* Vol. 2, No. 1, April, 1952, pp. 4-19. https://www.jstor.org/stable/1397459?seq=1#page_scan_tab_contents

H. B. Sprague. Emotional stress and the etiology of coronary heart disease. *Circulation.* Vol. 17, January, 1958, pp 1-4.

D. Summers. For the love of goop don't steam your vagina. *The Daily Beast.* January 29, 2015. https://www.thedailybeast.com/for-the-love-of-goop-dont-steam-your-vagina

The State of Obesity. *The healthcare costs of obesity.* https://www.stateofobesity.org/healthcare-costs-obesity/

J. Tilburt, MD, MPH, M. Allyse, PhD, and F. Hafferty, PhD. The case of Dr. Oz: Ethics, evidence, and does professional self-regulation work? *AMA Journal of Ethics.* February, 2017. https://journalofethics.ama-assn.org/article/case-dr-oz-ethics-evidence-and-does-professional-self-regulation-work/2017-02

Urban Dictionary. Insanity. https://www.urbandictionary.com/define.php?term=Insanity

T. VanderWeele, E. McNeely and H. Koh. Reimagining health – flourishing. *Journal of the American Medical Association.* April 1, 2019. https://jamanetwork.com/journals/jama/fullarticle/2730087

W. Wardwell & C. Behanson. Behavioural variables and MI in the Southeastern Connecticut Heart Study. *Journal of Chronic Diseases.* Vol. 26, 1973, pp. 447-461.

J. Weaver. More people search for health online: But they often can't find what they're looking for. *NBC News Online*. July 16, 2018. http://www.nbcnews.com/id/3077086/t/more-people-search-health-online/#.XEDN9VxKiUl

What is influencer marketing? *The Huffington Post*. July 5, 2015. https://www.huffingtonpost.com/global-yodel/what-is-influcner-marketing_b_10778128.html

D. Williamson and J. Carr. Health as a resource for everyday life: advancing the conceptualization. *Critical Public Health*. Vol. 19, 2009. https://www.tandfonline.com/doi/abs/10.1080/09581590802376234

L. Wilson. Sternberg's views on intelligence. *The Second Principle*. https://thesecondprinciple.com/optimal-learning/sternbergs-views-intelligence/

World Health Organization. The Ottawa Charter for Health Promotion First International Conference on Health Promotion, Ottawa, November 21, 1986. https://www.who.int/healthpromotion/conferences/previous/ottawa/en/

B. Zimmer. Wellness. *The New York Times*. April 16, 2010. https://www.nytimes.com/2010/04/18/magazine/18FOB-onlanguage-t.html

ABOUT THE AUTHOR

DR. ARTHUR H. PARSONS practiced family medicine and hypnotherapy for 45 years, 28 of those included a busy obstetrical practice. A graduate of the Dalhousie University School of Medicine in Halifax, Nova Scotia, Canada, Dr. Parsons was also a partner in Atlantic Offshore Medical Associates for 33 years, providing occupational health and medical services to offshore oil companies in the North Atlantic.

Some of his volunteer work in medical politics included ten years as the Chairman of Canadian Medical Association's Ethics Committee, and a term as a director for the Canadian Society of Medical Bioethics. He was also the president of the Canadian Association of Medical Clinics.

Dr. Parsons is the co-author of four previous health books including *Hippocrates Now! Is Your Doctor Ethical?* (University of Toronto Press) and *When Older is Wiser: A Guide to Healthcare Decisions for Older Adults and their Families* (Doubleday Canada). Dr. Parsons and his wife live in Toronto.

You can contact Dr. Parsons through MOONLIGHT PRESS

www.moonightpresstoronto.com

You can also connect with Dr. Parsons online:

TWITTER @lesshealthcare

INSTAGRAM @drarthurparsons

Parsons

Life is Terminal

Parsons

www.ingramcontent.com/pod-product-compliance
Lightning Source LLC
Chambersburg PA
CBHW030241030426
42336CB00009B/194